HEALTH AND HUMAN DEVELOPMENT

HEALTH PROMOTION

STRENGTHENING POSITIVE HEALTH AND PREVENTING DISEASE

HEALTH AND HUMAN DEVELOPMENT

JOAV MERRICK - SERIES EDITOR

NATIONAL INSTITUTE OF CHILD HEALTH
AND HUMAN DEVELOPMENT,
MINISTRY OF SOCIAL AFFAIRS, JERUSALEM

Adolescent Behavior Research: International Perspectives
Joav Merrick and Hatim A. Omar (Editors)
2007. ISBN: 1-60021-649-8

Complementary Medicine Systems: Comparison and Integration
Karl W. Kratky
2008. ISBN: 978-1-60456-475-4 (Hardcover)
2008. ISBN: 978-1-61122-433-7 (E-book)

Pain in Children and Youth
Patricia Schofield and Joav Merrick (Editors)
2008. ISBN: 978-1-60456-951-3 (Hardcover)
2008. ISBN: 978-1-61470-496-6 (E-book)

Children and Pain
Patricia Schofield and Joav Merrick (Editors)
2009. ISBN: 978-1-60876-020-6 (Hardcover)
2009. ISBN: 978-1-61728-183-9 (E-book)

Alcohol-Related Cognitive Disorders: Research and Clinical Perspectives
Leo Sher, Isack Kandel and Joav Merrick (Editors)
2009. ISBN: 978-1-60741-730-9 (Hardcover)
2009. ISBN: 978-1-60876-623-9 (E-book)

Challenges in Adolescent Health: An Australian Perspective
David Bennett, Susan Towns, Elizabeth Elliott and Joav Merrick (Editors)
2009. ISBN: 978-1-60741-616-6 (Hardcover)
2009. ISBN: 978-1-61668-240-8 (E-book)

Living on the Edge: The Mythical, Spiritual, and Philosophical Roots of Social Marginality
Joseph Goodbread
2009. ISBN: 978-1-60741-162-8 (Hardcover)
2013. ISBN: 978-1-61122-986-8 (Softcover)
2011. ISBN: 978-1-61470-192-7 (E-book)

Obesity and Adolescence: A Public Health Concern
Hatim A. Omar, Donald E. Greydanus, Dilip R. Patel and Joav Merrick (Editors)
2009. ISBN: 978-1-60692-821-9 (Hardcover)
2009. ISBN: 978-1-61470-465-2 (E-book)

Poverty and Children: A Public Health Concern
Alexis Lieberman and Joav Merrick (Editors)
2009. ISBN: 978-1-60741-140-6 (Hardcover)
2009. ISBN: 978-1-61470-601-4 (E-book)

Bone and Brain Metastases: Advances in Research and Treatment
Arjun Sahgal, Edward Chow and Joav Merrick (Editors)
2010. ISBN: 978-1-61668-365-8 (Hardcover)
2010. ISBN: 978-1-61728-085-6 (E-book)

Advanced Cancer Pain and Quality of Life
Edward Chow and Joav Merrick (Editors)
2011. ISBN: 978-1-61668-207-1 (Hardcover)
2010. ISBN: 978-1-61668-400-6 (E-book)

Chance Action and Therapy: The Playful Way of Changing
Uri Wernik
2010. ISBN: 978-1-60876-393-1 (Hardcover)
2011. ISBN: 978-1-61122-987-5 (Softcover)
2011. ISBN: 978-1-61209-874-6 (E-book)

Advances in Environmental Health Effects of Toxigenic Mold and Mycotoxins
Ebere Cyril Anyanwu
2011. ISBN: 978-1-60741-953-2

Alternative Medicine Yearbook 2009
Joav Merrick (Editor)
2011. ISBN: 978-1-61668-910-0 (Hardcover)
2011. ISBN: 978-1-62081-710-0 (E-book)

Behavioral Pediatrics, 3rd Edition
Donald E. Greydanus, Dilip R. Patel, Helen D. Pratt and Joseph L. Calles, Jr. (Editors)
2011. ISBN: 978-1-60692-702-1 (Hardcover)
2009. ISBN: 978-1-60876-630-7 (E-book)

Child Health and Human Development Yearbook 2009
Joav Merrick (Editor)
2011. ISBN: 978-1-61668-912-4

Climate Change and Rural Child Health
Erica Bell, Bastian M. Seidel and Joav Merrick (Editors)
2011. ISBN: 978-1-61122-640-9 (Hardcover)
2011. ISBN: 978-1-61209-014-6 (E-book)

Clinical Aspects of Psychopharmacology in Childhood and Adolescence
Donald E. Greydanus, Joseph L. Calles, Jr., Dilip P. Patel, Ahsan Nazeer and Joav Merrick (Editors)
2011. ISBN: 978-1-61122-135-0 (Hardcover)
2011. ISBN: 978-1-61122-715-4 (E-book)

Narratives and Meanings of Migration
Julia Mirsky
2011. ISBN: 978-1-61761-103-2 (Hardcover)
2010. ISBN: 978-1-61761-519-1 (E-book)

Drug Abuse in Hong Kong: Development and Evaluation of a Prevention Program
Daniel T.L. Shek, Rachel C.F. Sun and Joav Merrick (Editors)
2011. ISBN: 978-1-61324-491-3 (Hardcover)
2011. ISBN: 978-1-62257-232-8 (E-book)

Environment, Mood Disorders and Suicide
Teodor T. Postolache and Joav Merrick (Editors)
2011. ISBN: 978-1-61668-505-8 (Hardcover)
2011. ISBN: 978-1-62618-340-7 (E-book)

Human Development: Biology from a Holistic Point of View
Søren Ventegodt, Tyge Dahl Hermansen and Joav Merrick
2011. ISBN: 978-1-61470-441-6 (Hardcover)
2011. ISBN: 978-1-61470-541-3 (E-book)

International Aspects of Child Abuse and Neglect
Howard Dubowitz and Joav Merrick (Editors)
2011. ISBN: 978-1-60876-703-8 (Hardcover)
2010. ISBN: 978-1-61122-049-0 (Softcover)
2010. ISBN: 978-1-61122-403-0 (E-book)

Positive Youth Development: Implementation of a Youth Program in a Chinese Context
Daniel T.L Shek, Hing Keung Ma and Joav Merrick (Editors)
2011. ISBN: 978-1-61668-230-9 (Hardcover)

Positive Youth Development: Evaluation and Future Directions in a Chinese Context
Daniel T.L. Shek, Hing Keung Ma and Joav Merrick (Editors)
2011. ISBN: 978-1-60876-830-1 (Hardcover)
2011. ISBN: 978-1-62100-175-1 (Softcover)
2010. ISBN: 978-1-61209-091-7 (E-book)

Principles of Holistic Psychiatry: A Textbook on Holistic Medicine for Mental Disorders
Soren Ventegodt and Joav Merrick
2011. ISBN: 978-1-61761-940-3 (Hardcover)
2011. ISBN: 978-1-61122-263-0 (E-book)

Public Health Yearbook 2009
Joav Merrick (Editor)
2011. ISBN: 978-1-61668-911-7 (Hardcover)
2011. ISBN: 978-1-62417-365-3 (E-book)

Rural Child Health: International Aspects
Erica Bell and Joav Merrick (Editors)
2011. ISBN: 978-1-60876-357-3 (Hardcover)
2011. ISBN: 978-1-61324-005-2 (E-book)

Rural Medical Education: Practical Strategies
Erica Bell, Craig Zimitat and Joav Merrick (Editors)
2011. ISBN: 978-1-61122-649-2 (Hardcover)
2011. ISBN: 978-1-61209-476-2 (E-book)

Self-Management and the Health Care Consumer
Peter William Harvey
2011. ISBN: 978-1-61761-796-6 (Hardcover)
2011. ISBN: 978-1-61122-214-2 (E-book)

Sexology from a Holistic Point of View
Soren Ventegodt and Joav Merrick
2011. ISBN: 978-1-61761-859-8 (Hardcover)
2011. ISBN: 978-1-61122-262-3 (E-book)

Social and Cultural Psychiatry Experience from the Caribbean Region
Hari D. Maharajh and Joav Merrick (Editors)
2011. ISBN: 978-1-61668-506-5 (Hardcover)
2010. ISBN: 978-1-61728-088-7 (E-book)

The Dance of Sleeping and Eating among Adolescents: Normal and Pathological Perspectives
Yael Latzer and Orna Tzischinsky (Editors)
2011. ISBN: 978-1-61209-710-7 (Hardcover)
2011. ISBN: 978-1-62417-366-0 (E-book)

Understanding Eating Disorders: Integrating Culture, Psychology and Biology
Yael Latzer, Joav Merrick and Daniel Stein (Editors)
2011. ISBN: 978-1-61728-298-0 (Hardcover)
2011. ISBN: 978-1-61470-976-3 (Softcover)
2011. ISBN: 978-1-61942-054-0 (E-book)

Adolescence and Chronic Illness. A Public Health Concern
Hatim Omar, Donald E. Greydanus, Dilip R. Patel and Joav Merrick (Editors)
2012. ISBN: 978-1-60876-628-4 (Hardcover)
2010. ISBN: 978-1-61761-482-8 (E-book)

AIDS and Tuberculosis: Public Health Aspects
Daniel Chemtob and Joav Merrick (Editors)
2012. ISBN: 978-1-62081-382-9 (Softcover)
2012. ISBN: 978-1-62081-406-2 (E-book)

Alternative Medicine Yearbook 2010
Joav Merrick (Editor)
2012. ISBN: 978-1-62100-132-4 (Hardcover)
2011. ISBN: 978-1-62100-210-9 (E-book)

Alternative Medicine Research Yearbook 2011
Joav Merrick (Editor)
2012. ISBN: 978-1-62081-476-5 (Hardcover)
2012. ISBN: 978-1-62081-477-2 (E-book)

Applied Public Health: Examining Multifaceted Social or Ecological Problems and Child Maltreatment
John R. Lutzker and Joav Merrick (Editors)
2012. ISBN: 978-1-62081-356-0 (Hardcover)
2012. ISBN: 978-1-62081-388-1 (E-book)

Building Community Capacity: Minority and Immigrant Populations
Rosemary M Caron and Joav Merrick (Editors)
2012. ISBN: 978-1-62081-022-4 (Hardcover)
2012. ISBN: 978-1-62081-032-3 (E-book)

Building Community Capacity: Skills and Principles
Rosemary M Caron and Joav Merrick (Editors)
2012. ISBN: 978-1-61209-331-4 (Hardcover)
2012. ISBN: 978-1-62257-238-0 (E-book)

Child and Adolescent Health Yearbook 2009
Joav Merrick (Editor)
2012. ISBN: 978-1-61668-913-1 (Hardcover)
2012. ISBN: 978-1-62257-095-9 (E-book)

Child and Adolescent Health Yearbook 2010
Joav Merrick (Editor)
2012. ISBN: 978-1-61209-788-6 (Hardcover)
2012. ISBN: 978-1-62417-046-1 (E-book)

Child Health and Human Development Yearbook 2010
Joav Merrick (Editor)
2012. ISBN: 978-1-61209-789-3 (Hardcover)
2012. ISBN: 978-1-62081-721-6 (E-book)

Health Risk Communication
Marijke Lemal and Joav Merrick (Editors)
2013. ISBN: 978-1-62257-544-2 (Hardcover)
2012. ISBN: 978-1-62257-552-7 (E-book)

Human Immunodeficiency Virus (HIV) Research: Social Science Aspects
Hugh Klein and Joav Merrick (Editors)
2012. ISBN: 978-1-62081-293-8 (Hardcover)
2012. ISBN: 978-1-62081-346-1 (E-book)

Our Search for Meaning in Life: Quality of Life Philosophy
Søren Ventegodt and Joav Merrick
2012. ISBN: 978-1-61470-494-2 (Hardcover)
2011. ISBN: 978-1-61470-519-2 (E-book)

Public Health Yearbook 2010
Joav Merrick (Editor)
2012. ISBN: 978-1-61209-971-2
(Hardcover)
2012. ISBN: 978-1-62417-863-4
(E-book)

Public Health Yearbook 2011
Joav Merrick (Editor)
2012. ISBN: 978-1-62081-433-8
(Hardcover)
2012. ISBN: 978-1-62081-434-5
(E-book)

Randomized Clinical Trials and Placebo: Can You Trust the Drugs are Working and Safe?
Søren Ventegodt and Joav Merrick
2012. ISBN: 978-1-61470-067-8

The Astonishing Brain and Holistic Conciousness: Neuroscience and Vedanta Perspectives
Vinod D. Deshmukh
2012. ISBN: 978-1-61324-295-7

Translational Research for Primary Healthcare
Erica Bell, Gert. P. Westert and Joav Merrick (Editors)
2012. ISBN: 978-1-61324-647-4
(Hardcover)
2012. ISBN: 978-1-62417-409-4
(E-book)

Textbook on Evidence-Based Holistic Mind-Body Medicine: Basic Philosophy and Ethics of Traditional Hippocratic Medicine
Søren Ventegodt and Joav Merrick
2012. ISBN: 978-1-62257-052-2
(Hardcover)
2013. ISBN: 978-1-62257-707-1
(E-book)

Textbook on Evidence-Based Holistic Mind-Body Medicine: Basic Principles of Healing in Traditional Hippocratic Medicine
Søren Ventegodt and Joav Merrick
2012. ISBN: 978-1-62257-094-2
(Hardcover)
2012. ISBN: 978-1-62257-172-7
(E-book)

Textbook on Evidence-Based Holistic Mind-Body Medicine: Healing the Mind in Traditional Hippocratic Medicine
Søren Ventegodt and Joav Merrick
2012. ISBN: 978-1-62257-112-3
(Hardcover)
2012. ISBN: 978-1-62257-175-8
(E-book)

Textbook on Evidence-Based Holistic Mind-Body Medicine: Holistic Practice of Traditional Hippocratic Medicine
Søren Ventegodt and Joav Merrick
2012. ISBN: 978-1-62257-105-5 (Hardcover)
2012. ISBN: 978-1-62257-174-1 (E-book)

Textbook on Evidence-Based Holistic Mind-Body Medicine: Research, Philosophy, Economy and Politics of Traditional Hippocratic Medicine
Søren Ventegodt and Joav Merrick
2012. ISBN: 978-1-62257-140-6 (Hardcover)
2012. ISBN: 978-1-62257-171-0 (E-book)

Textbook on Evidence-Based Holistic Mind-Body Medicine: Sexology and Traditional Hippocratic Medicine
Søren Ventegodt and Joav Merrick
2012. ISBN: 978-1-62257-130-7 (Hardcover)
2012. ISBN: 978-1-62257-176-5 (E-book)

Treatment and Recovery of Eating Disorders
Daniel Stein and Yael Latzer (Editors)
2012. ISBN: 978-1-61470-259-7 (Hardcover)
2013. ISBN: 978-1-61470-259-7 (Softcover)

Adolescence and Sports
Dilip R. Patel, Donald E. Greydanus, Hatim Omar and Joav Merrick (Editors)
2013. ISBN: 978-1-60876-702-1 (Hardcover)
2010. ISBN: 978-1-61761-483-5 (E-book)

Alternative Medicine Research Yearbook 2012
Søren Ventegodt and Joav Merrick (Editors)
2013. ISBN: 978-1-62808-080-3

Building Community Capacity: Case Examples from Around the World
Rosemary M Caron and Joav Merrick (Editors)
2013. ISBN: 978-1-62417-175-8 (Hardcover)
2013. ISBN: 978-1-62417-176-5 (E-book)

Public Health Yearbook 2012
Joav Merrick (Editors)
2013. ISBN: 978-1-62808-078-0

Bullying: A Public Health Concern
Jorge C. Srabstein and Joav Merrick (Editors)
2013. ISBN: 978-1-62618-564-7 (Hardcover)
2013. ISBN: 978-1-62618-588-3 (E-book)

Conceptualizing Behavior in Health and Social Research: A Practical Guide to Data Analysis
Said Shahtahmasebi and Damon Berridge
2013. ISBN: 978-1-60876-383-2

Health and Happiness from Meaningful Work: Research in Quality of Working Life
Søren Ventegodt and Joav Merrick (Editors)
2013. ISBN: 978-1-60692-820-2 (Hardcover)
2013. ISBN: 978-1-61324-981-9 (E-book)

Health Promotion: Community Singing as a Vehicle to Promote Health
Jing Sun, Nicholas Buys and Joav Merrick (Editors)
2013. ISBN: 978-1-62618-908-9 (Softcover)

Living on the Edge: The Mythical, Spiritual, and Philosophical Roots of Social Marginality
Joseph Goodbread (Author)
2013. ISBN: 978-1-61122-986-8 (Softcover)

Managed Care in a Public Setting
Richard Evan Steele
2013. ISBN: 978-1-62417-970-9 (Softcover)
2013. ISBN: 978-1-62417-863-4 (E-book)

Pediatric and Adolescent Sexuality and Gynecology: Principles for the Primary Care Clinician
Hatim A. Omar, Donald E. Greydanus, Artemis K. Tsitsika, Dilip R. Patel and Joav Merrick (Editors)
2013. ISBN: 978-1-60876-735-9 (Softcover)

Advanced Cancer: Managing Symptoms and Quality of Life
Natalie Pulenzas, Breanne Lechner, Nemica Thavarajah, Edward Chow and Joav Merrick (Editors)
2013. ISBN: 978-1-62808-239-5 (Hardcover)
2013. ISBN: 978-1-62808-267-8 (E-book)

Health Promotion: Strengthening Positive Health and Preventing Disease

Jing Sun, Nicholas Buys and Joav Merrick (Editors)

2013. ISBN: 978-1-62257-870-2 (Hardcover)

2013. ISBN: 978-1-62808-621-8 (E-book)

HEALTH AND HUMAN DEVELOPMENT

HEALTH PROMOTION

STRENGTHENING POSITIVE HEALTH AND PREVENTING DISEASE

JING SUN, PH.D
NICHOLAS BUYS, PH.D
AND
JOAV MERRICK, M.D., M. MED. SC.,
D. M. SC.
EDITORS

New York

For permission to use material from this book please contact us:
Telephone 631-231-7269; Fax 631-231-8175
Web Site: http://www.novapublishers.com

Library of Congress Cataloging-in-Publication Data

Library of Congress Control Number: 2013944998

ISBN: 978-1-62257-870-2

Published by Nova Science Publishers, Inc. † New York

Contents

Introduction

Health promotion

Jing Sun, PhD*[*,1], Nicholas Buys, PhD[2] and Joav Merrick, MD, MMedSc, DMSc[3-6]

[1]School of Public Health and Griffith Health Institute, Griffith University, Gold Coast Campus, Queensland, Australia,
[2]Teaching and Learning, Griffith Health Executive, Griffith University, Gold Coast Campus,Queensland, Australia,
[3]National Institute of Child Health and Human Development, Jerusalem,
[4]Division of Pediatrics, Hadassah Hebrew University Medical Center, Mt Scopus Campus, Jerusalem,
[5]Office of the Medical Director, Health Services, Division for Intellectual and Developmental Disabilities, Ministry of Social Affairs and Social Services, Jerusalem, Israel and
[6]Kentucky Children's Hospital, University of Kentucky, Lexington, Kentucky, United States of America

The World Health Organization defines health promotion "as the process of enabling people to increase control over and to improve, their health". It moves beyond a focus on individual behaviour towards a wide range of social

[*] *Correspondence:* Jing Sun, PhD, School of Public Health and Griffith Health Institute, Griffith University, Gold Coast Campus, Parkland, Southport, QLD 4222, Australia. E-mail: j.sun@griffith.edu.au

and environmental interventions, but discussions on how to define health promotion already emerged in the 1970s from the Lalonde report in Canada, which contained a health promotion strategy "aimed at informing, influencing and assisting both individuals and organizations so that they will accept more responsibility and be more active in matters affecting mental and physical health".

Health promotion and health service using socio-ecological approach has been effective to promote mental, physical health, improve social functioning and social support in a range of population group. Socio-ecological approach addresses the importance of the interaction between individual level characteristics, families, institutions, and community support to promote health to optimal level.

There is an increasing evidence to indicate promoting resilience at both individual and organisation levels is important to help with individuals to cope daily stress, challenges, and buffer the adverse effects of distress, abuse and neglect, psychological traumatic events, and diseases. The key concepts of resilience promotion is structured around self-esteem, self-efficacy, optimistic, goal orientation, autonomy, and ability to seek social and environmental support. These concepts play important role in improve quality of life, chronic disease conditions, increasing exercise level, and reduction of risk health behaviours.

In this special issue, we provide evidence to demonstrate the central concepts of health promotion around resilience at individual and organisation and system level is important to children's and youth quality of life, their learning outcomes, benefit employees' performance and health outcome, and chronic disease, dental student stress, depression and anxiety, and dental patients' knowledge about treatment and their health outcomes.

SECTION ONE: CHALLENGES

In: Health Promotion
Editors: J. Sun, N. Buys, J. Merrick

ISBN: 978-1-62257-870-2

Chapter I

Challenges, opportunities and strategies in mental health promotion in China: Literature review of mental health promotion models

***Jing Sun, PhD**[*1] **and Nicholas Buys, PhD**[2]*
[1]School of Public Health and Griffith Health Institute, Griffith University, Gold Coast Campus, Parkland, Gold Coast, Australia
[2]School of Human Services and Social Work, and Griffith Health Institute, Griffith University, Parkland, Gold Coast, Australia

Abstract

This chapter reviews the issue of high levels of mental health problems among Chinese children. It argues that current strategies used to address these problems are inadequate. As an alternative it explores the potential for a socio-ecological approach, focussed on mental health promotion and prevention, to address resilience—an emerging area to promote mental health. A key insight in this chapter is that mental health is determined by

[*] *Correspondence:* Jing Sun, PhD, School of Public Health, Griffith University and Griffith Health Institute, Griffith University, Gold Coastcampus, Parkland, Q4222 Australia. E-mail: j.sun@griffith.edu.au.

not only qualities of the individual child (i.e., cognitive and social competences) but also the characteristics of the systems in which children develop (i.e., a good sense of connectedness to family, peers and school community). The socio-ecological model, focussing on building children's skills, and placing greater emphasis on changing contexts and strengthening relationships, is seen as an effective approach to improve children's resilience, hence mental health. It is suggested that the socio-ecological approach should be used more widely in China to improve children's resilience and social and emotional wellbeing.

Introduction

In 1948, the World Health Organisation defined health as a 'state of complete physical, mental and social wellbeing and not merely the absence of disease of infirmity' (1). Unfortunately, this visionary conception did not guide research or service delivery in human health in China. Instead, the past half century showed a persistent focus on health from an illness and disease perspective, ignoring issues of psychological and social wellness. For example, during the period 1950 to 1990, public health efforts mainly focused on effective control of fatal communicable and infectious diseases, severe endemic diseases, severe infectious diarrhoea, infant pneumonia, and high morbidity and mortality caused by severe malnutrition. There is no doubt that this focus has resulted in a dramatic decrease in infant mortality and morbidity rates (2). However, we argue that mental health and social and emotional well-being should now be major components of health delivery, especially given the decline in communicable and infectious diseases in the more developed social-economic areas of China.

Current issues

The burden of mental health problems appears to be increasing in China, adversely affect individuals, families and communities. This increase is associated with the rapid social and economic development and changes that have taken place over recent years (3). Mental health problems in China now rank fourth in morbidity after diseases such as cardiac diseases, diabetes, and cancer (4). Suicide, in association with depression, is now the primary cause of death for youth, with an increasing incidence in lower age groups as well. (5).

The incidence of students who have mental health problems is now 16.4% for primary school students, and 14.2% for secondary school students (6).

Mental health issues for Chinese children relate to social and emotional problems and inability to adapt change and challenges (7). Poor relationships between children and parents and students and teachers compound feelings of loneliness and anxiety, and exacerbate hostile behaviour in children (7,8). However, such issues remain largely neglected as priorities for mental health service delivery, Considering the large youth population in China and the heavy burden on family and society of childhood mental health problems, this situation can no longer be ignored,

Traditional treatment and therapy, such as clinical psychological diagnosis and treatment, behavioural therapy, and individual education programs, do not effectively deal with many of these problems. Although scientific advances have led to aetiological discoveries and improved diagnostic tools, thereby reducing the severity and number of mental health problems (3), this has not led to the widespread alleviation of suffering. Clinical services provided by Chinese Mental Health Research Centers (i.e., the Child Mental Health Research Center in Nanjing) are limited due to the overwhelming numbers of people who require assistance. Efforts to prevent mental health problems and promote mental health and well-being have received little recognition in society. Prevention therefore remains an unrealised tool in China.

Causes of mental health problems in Chinese children

One of the ongoing debates in the literature has focused on whether the criteria to measure adaptation should include *both* internal adaptation and daily challenges (positive psychological well-being versus distress, depression, and anxiety) and external adaptation to changing environment and various cultural contexts. This debate reflects the dual nature of living systems (9,10). Human individuals are living organisms that must maintain coherence as a unit and also function as part of larger systems, such as families, communities, and society. From a perspective that views children's developmental success as grounded in the surrounding social conditions of their development, the fact that a significant number of children are not doing well in terms of their academic achievement, social and behavioural choices, and mental health suggests serious problems not only within children themselves but also across the broader cast of adults, families, institutions and policy context charged with helping them become full members of society. This was the view of Erikson (11) who believed that successful identity development in children involves the overall configuration of ego needs and the social ethos and contexts of families, schools and communities during a particular moment in life. The quality of fit between the developmental needs of children and the nature of the social opportunities afforded them by adults and communities may provide answers to the question of why some Chinese adolescents have academic, social, and emotional success, whereas a substantial minority of young Chinese children do not.

The problems facing millions of Chinese children are rooted in debilitating social and environmental conditions that include poor school organisational structures, overly demanding school curricula, inadequate mental health services, insufficient focus on social and emotional development, loneliness and anxiety due to the lack of peer interactions, high expectations from parents and society, and the absence of after-school and community recreational programs for children (12,13). Such conditions undermine the fulfilment of basic children and adolescent physical and physiological development needs (e.g., play, leisure, and safety) and also their basic psychological needs for trusting and accepting relationships with adults and peers, for self-expression and exploration, and for developing their academic and social competencies in the direction of viable occupational and social outcomes (11).

Often the key criterion of judgement of success for a young person in China is to graduate from university and gain the education and occupational skills needed for financial independence. In line with cultural traditions, children are also expected by their parents to outperform their peers in terms of academic achievement. In order to fulfil their expectations, parents invest their time, energy, money and intellect in the development of the one child, often neglecting their specific personal interests, talents and feelings. School curricula is often arranged to prepare children for examinations, rather than being centred on the developmental needs of the child. Resilient children and youth manage to meet these expectations, even though they may have faced more significant obstacles to success in life than children in most developed countries. However, the increasing numbers of children who have social, emotional and mental problems indicate that they are not able to cope, and therefore require a substantial support from health, psychological and social services.

Emerging area to promote children's mental health

In research relating to children over the past three decades,the concept ofresilience has emerged from the studies on individuals who adapt to extraordinary circumstances, achieving positive and unexpected outcomes in the face of adversity (9, 14). Resilience is inferred because two major judgements are required to identify individuals as belonging in this class of phenomena. First, individuals are judged as to whether they are 'doing OK' or 'better than OK' with respect to a set of expectations for behaviour and second, they are judged as to they thrive even when there have been extenuating circumstances that posed a threat their good outcomes. For example, some children survive without developing serious problems even though they are exposed to hostile environments (15). Resilient children seem to have a self-correcting capacity, an ability to respond with resourcefulness and tenacity when confronted with challenges or adversity. Resilience is a dynamic response to a multiplex of biological, psychological, social, and other environmental influences. For children, resilience is closely tied to development. The skills and competence that characterise resilient functioning at one point in time may thrive in the face of new developmental challenges or new contingencies in the environment.

Studies on school-aged children's positive development have found that children who develop well have several variables in common. These include, firstly, good *internal strengths*, such as sufficient personal assets and competencies, high self-esteem, an internal locus of control, optimism and clear aspirations, achievement and goal-orientation, reflectiveness and problem solving capacity, respect for the autonomy of themselves and others, and healthy communication patterns. Secondly, they include effective *external nurturance and support* from the social environment, such as nurturing and supportive family, school and community environments. These resources, recognised as protective factors, contribute to their positive development and protect them from stress and dysfunction (10,14). Protective factors are "the quality of persons or contexts that predict better outcomes under high-risk conditions" (10). Protective factors predict future outcomes. Protective factors modify risk by directly reducing a disorder or dysfunction, and they mediate risk in chains of risk and protective factors (16). Sometimes, too, they provide resistance to risk by moderating the relationship among risk factors and problems or disorders (17). The latter usually is called a "buffering" effect, because it buffers an individual against the full effect of risk. Protective factors are important because they provide clues for designing more effective social programs. They identify potentially targetable influences that, if fostered by a program, may directly affect a problem or moderate a risk related to a problem (18). Protective factors that refer to individual characteristics (i.e., an easy-going temperament, high self-esteem and self-efficacy) are often recognised as human capital or personal strength. Group or community factors, such as family factors (i.e., parental warmth and supervision), or extra-familial conditions (i.e., having a network of supportive friends) are often referred to as components of social capital in the resilience literature (10,14).

Mental health effects from individual characteristics

Individual characteristics allow the option of maximizing opportunities in the context of personal limitations and environmental adversity. Generally, individuals characteristics include positive psychological characteristics, such as positive affection and emotion, high self-esteem, and competent social emotional abilities, tend to be physically, socially, and mentally active (19). Also, contemporary researchers emphasise that it is the process of striving for goals—rather than goal attainment *per se*—that is crucial for positive psychological development (19). Myers and Diener (20) conclude that satisfaction with life grows from involvement in valued activities and progress toward one's goal rather than from passive experience of desirable circumstances. Following this argument, it is essential that we perceive these things to be important and as representing goals that are well worth pursuing. The details of mental health effects from individual characteristics, such as, positive affection and emotion, high self-esteem, optimism, and self-efficacy, are discussed below.

Positive affection and emotion

Experiencing positive emotions such as joy, interest, contentment, love, and the like significantly contribute to optimal functioning. Experiments on humans and animals found that positive traits and states and behaviours linked with positive states-such as play –lead to increases in physical, intellectual, and social resources. Furthermore, positive emotions also produce improved well-being. For example, if positive emotions broaden the scope of cognition and enable flexible and creative thinking, they also should facilitate coping with stress and adversity. By broadening people's modes of thinking and action, positive emotions should improve coping and thus build resilience. Increments in resilience should in turn, predict future experiences of positive emotions (21).

Self-esteem

In resilience research on human strengths, self-esteem is thought of as a sign of well-being for two reasons. First, reasonably good self-esteem provides an indication that mood is working within optimal limits to motivate and caution human action. Self-esteem is a measure of the person's expectation of positive events, and accordingly, her or his willingness to approach objects and others. Second, and more broadly, good self-esteem is indicative of a positive and integral personal and social identity (22)—that is, a sense that one is located securely in the social world, competent to meet its challenges, ready to participate in life with others, and able to balance social demands and personal desires. Effective ways to achieve good self-esteem must recognise a number of conditions, namely: acceptance within a social context, a sense of security, cultural competence, and the capacity to reconcile personal goals and social expectations. Hewitt (23) proposed that the individual and the good of the community should be reconciled. Individuals are products of their community but also its creators. When people experience self-esteem, they are living in the affective link between individual and community.

Optimism

Optimism is the expectation people have that good things will happen to them. Studies on optimism found that optimists experience less distress than pessimists when dealing with difficulties in their lives. People who are confident about the future exert continuing effort, even when dealing with serious adversity (24). Optimists use more problem-centred coping than pessimists. They also used a variety of emotion-focused coping techniques, including working to accept the reality for difficult situations and putting the situations in the best possible light. These findings indicate that optimists may have a coping advantage over pessimists even in situations that cannot be changed.

Self-efficacy

Self-efficacy is defined as beliefs about the ability to attain desired goals in particular domains and circumstances. It is not concerned with beliefs about the ability to perform specific and trivial motor acts but with beliefs about ability to coordinate and orchestrate skills and abilities in changing and challenging situations. Self-efficacy is influenced primarily by two interacting factors. First, it is influenced by the development of the capacity for symbolic thought, particularly the capacity for understanding cause-and-effect relationships and the capacity for self-observation and self-reflection. Children must learn that one event can cause another event; that they are separate from other things and people; and that, they can be the origin of actions that affect their environment.

Second, self-efficacy is influenced by the responsiveness of the environment, especially social environments, to the infant or child's attempts at manipulation and control. Environments that are responsive to the child's actions facilitate the development of efficacy beliefs, whereas nonresponsive environments impair this development. Thus, children usually develop a sense of efficacy from engaging in actions that manipulate the people around them, which then generalizes to the non-social environment (25). Parents can facilitate or hinder the development of this sense of efficacy not only by their response to the infant's or child's actions, but also by encouraging and enabling the child to explore and master his or her environment. A sense of control over our behaviour, our environment, and our own thoughts and feelings is essential for happiness and a sense of well-being, together with meeting life's challenges, building healthy relationships, and achieving personal satisfaction and peace of mind.

Mental health effects from social capital

Social capital is related to family and community support and structure that promote personal competence including self-esteem, self-efficacy, problem solving, or providing guidance at points of life transition.

A school's social climate, reflected in the sense of connectedness to others and support from the social environment, are well-established correlates of resilience and contribute to numerous positive outcomes for children (26). The sense of the positive classroom climate affected school satisfaction directly and indirectly through its influence on stress and psychological distress. For example in the Baker et al (27) study, classroom environments that are perceived as friendly, supportive and free of harassment, are associated with school satisfaction and perceived quality of teacher-student relationships from both teacher and child perspectives. This also predicts student school-related outcomes and behaviours (28). The teacher-student relationship has been identified as a significant influence on overall school and behavioral adjustment (28). Teachers who "provide emotional support, reward competence, and promote self-esteem" (p.10) are considered to be one of the factors that decrease the vulnerability of high-risk students in response to stressful life events (29).

Classroom structures, goals, and practices

Specific classroom practices are associated with positive school attitudes (30). Tasks that provide optimal levels of challenge, feedback that is informational rather than judgemental, recognition of mastery efforts rather than relative performance, and minimisation of interpersonal competition, are all associated with enhanced academic motivation. Classroom practices that afford students opportunities to feel competent and to exercise developmentally appropriate autonomy are associated with a positive appraisal of school. Some developmental models of school reform afford a view of the linkages between school practices and positive school attitudes.

Peer influence

Children's peers play an important role in their positive development and wellness. Friendships serve as an important context for students' comfort and support and have been considered an important part of social context for human development (31). Peer groups also serve to socialize children, causing them to adopt similar goals and attitudes to their peers. Wentzel (32) found that children who felt their peers supported them, adopted prosocial and socially responsible goals within the classroom, such as aiding classmates in classroom activities. In contrast, socially rejected adolescents who are actively disliked by many peers perceive less social support within the classroom and exhibit less positive psychosocial, behavioural, and academic outcomes. Some evidence suggests a link between peer relationships and a sense of school connectedness. Chen et al (31) found that Chinese students in China who had more friends and had high quality of friendships have more positive attitudes toward school, school-related competence, and academic achievement. As in the classroom climate area, social contexts that are characterised by positive attitudes and lack negative ones are associated with increased school satisfaction.

Family influence

The influence of the family is pervasive on children's development. For example, home environment predicts significant positive changes in children's overall adjustment (33), and predicts increased positive expectations for the future (34). Specifically, families influence positive adaptation in many ways including modelling academically oriented behaviours, socializing an achievement orientation and values regarding education, and direct teaching and structuring of the home so that school tasks are prioritised, emphasized and accommodated (35). The active involvement of home with schools provides continuity across these two critical developmental settings and extends opportunities for learning activities outside of school (36)). Parental involvement in school has been found to be a better predictor of school adjustment and engagement, and children's well-being than other measures of parenting behaviour including monitoring and expectations (36). This probably is because parents demonstrate their care and concern for the children and provide opportunities for direction and encouragement by knowing a lot about the life of their children.

In summary, it can be concluded that there are two effects deriving from the protective factors discussed above. The first effect is a compensatory protective effect, typically directly reducing a problem or disorder. One usually think of a compensatory protective effects as a statistical main effect. That is, it does not affect risk but rather exerts a direct effect on a problem or disorder. In a study of over 36,000 seventh-through 12th grade students in Minnesota, compensatory protective effects for externalising problem behaviours were found for family, school connectedness, plus low exposure to poverty, parental unemployment, parental substance abuse, and domestic violence (37). Werner (38) identified protective factors which included significant relationships with kin, intimate partners, and mentors, such as coaches or teachers, who supported their efforts, believed in their potential, and encouraged them to make the most of their lives. Wolin and Wolin (39) identified seven protective factors which included insight, independence, fulfilling relationships, initiative, creativity, humour, and the capacity to distinguish good from bad. These are conceptualised as directly altering the chances of negative future outcomes.

The second effect of protective factors is interactional. With the advance of more complex conceptualisation of protective factors, Rutter (14) proposed that the developmental outcome of a human is whole person and behaviour as a function of person in interaction with environment. He has argued that protective factors are defined both by compensatory effects and perhaps more importantly, by interactional effects i.e. those effect that moderate risk. This interactional perspective does not exclude a possibility that a factor exerts an important influence on people who are not at risk. To be an interactional protective effect, a factor must exert an even stronger, positive effect on children who have been exposed to adversity.

Unlike research in vulnerability, which focuses on children in high-risk settings, the study of resilience encompasses all children and focuses on positive development. It has been found that the socio-ecological model with its orientation towards to community development to enhance child outcomes and focus on building positive adjustments in children allows for new insight into mental health promotion amongst young people in China. As a 'settings' approach to health promotion, it has the potential to promote resilience since it is based on the inclusive, participatory and democratic principles shown to be necessary for the development of resilience at the broader community level. The model illustrates this potential through two mechanisms. The first is **processes** that are characterised by inclusivity and the meaningful, active participation of the diverse range of members that make up a school community as well as equal 'power' relationships, or equal partnerships among community members, parents and school staff. The second are **structural mechanisms** such as school policies, school organisation and the school's physical environment; reflect the values of participation, democracy and inclusiveness and/or that promote processes based on these values. These processes and structures typified by the socio-ecological model, and located in the broad school environment and the immediate classroom environment collectively have potential to promote resilience in the school setting.

Social ecological framework to promote mental health

The theoretical development of mental health promotion research is underpinned by the notion that mental health is the transactional product of individual attributes and environmental contingencies. Adaptational response is often tied to skills and competences in problem solving, interpersonal attributes, coping, as well as an ability to act in a planned way. Such attributes are considered to be core elements of resilience (40), but they also interact with and often depend on familial and extra-familial resources. Because the contexts in which individual develop play an influential role in promoting their adaptation and adjustment (26), the degree to which schools function as psychologically healthy environments is a key issue within resilience research as applied to children.

The Social Ecological Model draws on this notion. For example, a fundamental concept of this model is that being autonomous and in a position to choose to function well is necessary to maximise health potential. It follows from this fundamental concept that the promotion of health is facilitated by the promotion of student functioning. The primary mechanisms through which schools promote student resilience and hence health, are through the influence of school system including school organisation, curriculum development, and educational practices on pupil development. This notion is supported by a variety of World Health Organization documents that argue that in order to promote health, the health promotions needs to shift from focusing on the modification of individual risk factors or risk behavior to addressing the "context and meaning" of health actions and the determinants that keep people healthy. School as a health promoting setting should not neglect their management structures, internal and external relationships as well as teaching and learning (41). Others support this focus arguing that in order to be health promoting, social institutions such as schools should focus on their organisational systems and human interaction within the organisation (42,43).

The Social Ecological framework is multidisciplinary, using a population based approach which acknowledges the range of influences on mental health and wellbeing. These include biological, psychological and social factors and more broadly, their interactions with environmental and economic factors (44). Unlike research on psychoanalytic or behavioral therapy which focuses on the diagnosis, deficiency treatment and illness therapy of individuals, the socio-ecological approach focuses on the prevention of mental health problems and early intervention to promote mental health and well-being. It emphasises building up individual and community strengths and capacity to respond with resourcefulness and tenacity in the face of adversity and challenges. The socio ecological health promotion Model specifically addresses: social determinants of health, enhancement of human capital, and enhancement of social capital.

Social ecological health promotion model and social determinants of health

The socio ecological health promotion approach has been proven to be effective at aggregate, population or community levels of action (45-47). By focusing on the settings where people congregate, lead their daily lives and interact on a regular basis, health promotion professionals can work with communities to help create environments that positively affect the behavior that occurs in the setting, and intervene to create change in aspects of those settings that foster behavior with negative consequences. Within these perspectives, children are seen as genetic contributors to their own development. As they interact with social settings, children construct meaning about themselves, others and the nature of school. The meanings children derive from the environment influence their beliefs about themselves as individuals, as learners, and about the purpose, nature and goals of those that they meet in the school and the formal educational processes that take place. These beliefs, in turn, affect children's engagement and participation in school. The school thus influences development because their climate characteristics affect children's appraisals of the school environment, their sense of belonging and connectedness. This in turn affects children's cognition about school, their school-related behaviours, and hence well-being (48). For example, practices that extend a sense of classroom community are likely to be appraised as supportive by students, resulting in increased satisfaction and school engagement (27). Schools also directly affect development because their structure and practices exert a socialising influence on student. For example, there are significant differences in school attitudes and academic outcomes between students in academic and non-academic "tracks", suggesting that educational practice may be a significant factor associated with student's differential outcomes.

Schools are likely to have a positive influence on children's development if there is a good fit between the developmental needs of students and the school environment. Self-determination theory may be used to guide the understanding of student's needs. This theory posits that individuals have three fundamental developmental needs: to be meaningfully connected to others, to have developmentally appropriate choice and self-direction, and to perceive themselves as competent in their endeavours (49). Schools that afford opportunities for students to satisfy these needs would promote student health and well-being (43).

Promotion of individual characteristics

The notion that individual characteristics can be enhanced is based on the assumption that the power of human adaptational systems can be mobilized. These strategies aim to mobilize fundamental protective systems for development. Efforts have been made to influence processes that will change a child's life rather than simply remove risk or adding assets. In terms of increasing the sense of connectedness within the school environment there is good evidence to indicate that this promotes mental and emotional well-being (50-52) and is protective against health risk-taking behaviours related to substance use, violence and early sexual behaviour (51,53). Evidence also indicates that a sense of belonging and connectedness also contributes to improved academic achievement and engagement (50,54,55) as well as to reducing crime (56, 57). As a significant protective factor for several health, academic and social outcomes, school connectedness has enormous potential to contribute to child and adolescent health and development into adulthood (58-60).

A wide range of programs have been designed to improve the quality of attachment and build self-esteem, self-efficacy to succeed in life, such as the Social and Emotional Learning program in New Haven, Connecticut, public schools (61), and the Resolving Conflict Creatively Program (RCCP) that began in the New York city public schools (62). The program goals include increasing awareness of the different choices available to children for dealing with conflicts; developing skills for making these choices, encouraging children's respect for their own cultural background and the background of others; teaching children how to identify and stand against prejudice; and increasing children's awareness of their role in creating a more peaceful world. A follow-up program, Peace in the Family, trains parents in conflict resolution strategies.

Promotion of social capital

The notion that the social capital can be built up is on the basis of the assumption that the number or quality of resources or social capital can be improved and that whilst the human capital conceptualisations recognise the importance of individual attributes associated with resilience, the school as a social institution involves multiple actors and agencies. The notion of social capital helps to remind us of the importance of links to other social systems such as the family environment and the broader community environment, including health services and community agencies, that have an enormous impact on the health of children and adolescents within the school (63) and on the effectiveness of the school as an educational institution (64-67).

It has been argued that a clearer insight into the nature of school connectedness can be provided by conceiving it as an ecological concept (68). This allows a more complete recognition of the nature and associated processes of the school environment and recognises valuable social systems such as the family environment and the broader community. These systems influence on the health of children and adolescents and on the general effectiveness of the school.

In China, the school context can be understood as: competition for places, stern teaching style, and strict classroom control. Although more than 20% of students can have the opportunity to go to university, the struggle in Chinese society for school success and employment is intense nowadays. The pressure to succeed is relentless and exerts a considerable toll in student anxiety and depression, not to mention family pressure around the doing of homework. Class sizes are large because resources are often scarce, but more importantly because the Chinese believe that "on one mountain, there cannot be two tigers", in other words, competition will better enable the best student to get to the top, thereby proving that the best choice has been made. There is little opportunity for individual instruction in class, examinations are frequent and grading is based almost exclusively on their outcomes. Students respond to teachers as to a stern parent—with attention, silence, and fear. They do not question teachers, or challenge their judgements. In classroom, great amounts of time are devoted to academic activities, and most of the class time is devoted to activities where the teacher is in charge. Such a school context is opposite against to the notion of resilience and the socio ecological approach outlined above.

From socio ecological theoretical perspective, a teachers' perception of their own ability to handle challenging behaviours and to establish positive relationships has a possible influence on the quality of teacher-student relationship. High teacher self-efficacy and low teacher stress has been linked to a variety of positive outcomes, such as positive classroom environments, and better relationships with students (28).

Positive peer relationships provide an avenue to meet student's developmental needs for connectedness to others, thus enhancing their positive adjustment and well-being at school. Children in China are generally discouraged from participating in informal peer groups because they may threaten adults' authority. Parents and teachers may be particularly concerned about negative influences of deviant peers and thus likely exert high control and supervision on children's peer groups (69). Evidence indicates that the percentage of students in Chinese schools (70%) involved in peer groups is substantially lower than what is typically reported in Western cultures (about 85-90%) (70).

Studies examining the antecedents and determinants of the quality of school life have also explored mental health variables such as self-esteem, depression, and stress.

Due to the scarcity of the quality of school life literature in China, examining mental health variables associated with life satisfaction from western research is useful. Research suggests there are strong interrelationships between psychological and environmental variables that influence quality of school life.

For instance, Baker (27) found that school climate had a significant indirect effect on school satisfaction by influencing psychological variables such as psychological distress and self-concept. Furthermore, internal locus of control mediated the relationship between negative life experiences and quality of school life, indicating the contribution of both psychological and environmental variables to quality of school life. The interplay of these variables implies the necessity of optimising many aspects of children's lives in order to promote their quality of school life.

Social ecological framework and Chinese child mental health

We have argued that the school environment and climate does not seem to meet students' psychological needs in China. School systems in China will clearly need to change or be modified if they are on the one hand to help promote mental health and well-being yet, on the other hand remain true to cultural characteristics. The increasing level of mental illness amongst young people is a pressing and significant problem, and prevention efforts must be prioritised in order to limit and reduce the impact of this problem. The socio ecological approach uses a comprehensive methodology which allows for multi-strategy efforts to address the problem. Such efforts will be mutually supportive and involve all those with whom young people come into contact in the school setting. This approach may help China to solve a number of mental health problems that students, family and school community currently confront.

An orientation toward positive development and building on strengths has significant implications for research using a social ecological approach in China. This perspective challenges China to consider markers of positive adjustment rather than diagnosis of developmental problems and to engage in preventative rather than reactive models of practice. Considering not just the prevention of dysfunction but the promotion of adjustment is a critical feature of socio ecological approach to school-based practice. This type of research recognises the reality of health as an integral part of everyday life, and the added complexities when studying the influence of environmental features.

China's economic development poses a challenge to the thousand year tradition of the Confucian family where the role of the person is fundamentally to submit and adapt. As China continue to modernise, Chinese people are facing with the challenge of serving both as a force and recipient of change in their social world, including larger society, school community, family unit and individual. As this change will occur at varying speeds for different members and in different context, what once was a more static social world is likely to become more dynamic, changing and challenging. These challenges have brought already and will inevitably bring about disequilibration for the individual, family and community, and propose an essential question for the mental health of Chinese peoples.

Environments are complex in China, and include multifaceted entities that create numerous theoretical difficulties for research. Careful conceptual analysis of the potentially reciprocal, hierarchical, and embedded nature of relationships between children, school, community and social environments need to be considered. Despite these concerns, it is believed that socio ecological approach has an important place in the research of Chinese children's resilience and mental health. The perspectives that development is transactional and that environments play key roles in shaping or constraining development are important as theory unfolds in this area. The sensitivity to the effects of socio ecological approach on children's development encourages us to look critically and creatively at environmental contributors to Chinese children's resilience.

References

[1] WHO. World Health Organisation constitution. Geneva: 1948.

[2] Zhu ZH. Strengthen micro-health concepts and draw up the plan of prevention and health in new millennium. China Hospital Management 1998;14(6):322-6.

[3] Zhou Y, Yang X, eds. Second Sino-American mental health conference. 2000; Beijing, China.

[4] Murray CJL, Lopez AD. Global mortality, disability, and the contribution of risk factors: Global burden of disease study. Lancet 1997;349(1436-42).

[5] Parker G, Gladstone G, Chee KT. Depression in the planet's largest ethnic group: The Chinese. Am J Psychiatry 2001;158(6):857-64.

[6] Liu X, Kurita H, Guo C, Miyake Y, Ze J, Cao H. Prevalence and risk factors of behavioral and emotional problems among Chinese children aged 6 through 11 year. J Am Acad Child Adolesc Psychol 1999;38(6):708-71.

[7] Yang B, Ollendick TH, Dong Q, Xia Y, Lin L. Only children and children with siblings in the People's Republic of China: Levels of fear, anxiety, and depression. Child Dev 1995;66:1301-11.

[8] Liu X, Sun Z, Neiderhiser JM, Uchiyama M, Okawa M, Rogan W. Behavioral and emotional problems in Chinese adolescents: Parent and teacher reports. J Am Acad Child Adolesc Psychiatr 2001;40(7):828-36.

[9] Masten AS, Coatsworth JD. Competence, resilience, and psychopathology. In: Cicchetti. D, Cohen. D, eds. Developmental psychopathology. New York: Wiley, 1995:715-52.

[10] Masten AS, Reed MJ. Resilience in development. In: Snyder CR, Lopez SJ, eds. Handbook of positive psychology. New York: Oxford University Press, 2002: 74-88.

[11] Erikson EH. Identity, youth and crisis. New York: Norton, 1968.

[12] Chen Y. Chinese classification of mental disorders (CCMD-3): Towards integration in international classification. Psychopathology 2002;35:171-5.

[13] Ying YW, Zhang X. Mental health in rural and urban families: The role of intergenerational personality discrepancy and family solidarity. J Comparative Fam Stud 1995;26(2):233-9.

[14] Rutter M. Psychosocial resilience and protective mechanisms. Am J Orthopsychiatry 1987;57:316-31.

[15] Smith CA, Lizotte AJ, Thornberry TP, Krohn MD. Resilience to delinquency. Prev Res 1997;4(2):4-7.

[16] Coie JD, Watt NF, West SG, Hawkins JD, Asarnow JR, Markman HJ, et al. The science of prevention: A conceptual framework and some directions for a National Research Program. Am Psychol 1993;48:1013-22.

[17] Bryant KJ, West SG, Windle M. Overview of new methodological developments in prevention research: Alcohos and substance abuse. In: Bryant. KJ, Windle. M, S. G. W, eds. The science of prevention: Methodological advances from alcohol and substance abuse research. Washington, DC: American Psychological Association, 1997:xvii-xxxii.

[18] Burt MR, Resnick G, Novick ER. Building supportive communities for at-risk adolescents: it takes more than services. Washington, DC: American Psychological Association, 1998.

[19] Watson D. Mood and temperament. New York: Guilford, 2000.

[20] Myers DG, Diener E. Who is happy? Psychol Sci 1995;6:10-9.

[21] Fredrickson BL. Positive emotions. In: Snyder. CR, Lopez SJ, editors. Handbook of Positive Psychology. Oxford: Oxford University Press, 2002:120-34.

[22] Hewitt JP. The myth of self-esteem: Finding happiness and solving problems in American. New York: St. Martin's, 1998.

[23] Hewitt JP. The social construction of self-esteem. In: Snyder. CR, Lopez. SJ, eds. Handbook of positive psychology. Oxford: Oxford University Press, 2002:135-47.

[24] Carver CS, Scheier MF. Optimism. In: Snyder CR, Lopez SJ, eds. Handbook of positive psychology. Oxford: Oxford University Press, 2002:231-43.

[25] Bandura A. Self-efficacy: The exercise of control. New York: Freeman, 1997.

[26] Masten A, Best KM, Garmezy N. Resiliency and development: Contributions from the study of children who overcome adversity. Dev Psychopathol 1991;2:425-44.

[27] Baker JA. Teacher-student interaction in urban "at-risk" classrooms; Differential behaviour, relationship quality, and student satisfaction with school. Jf Elementary Educ 1999;100:57-70.

[28] Yoon JS. Teacher characteristics as predictors of teacher-student relationships: Stress, negative affect, and self-efficacy. Soc Behav Pers 2002;30(5):485-93.

[29] Werner EE. Protective factors and individual resilience. In: Meisels. SJ, Shonkoff. JP, eds. Handbook of early childhood intervention. New York: Cambridge University Press, 1990:97-116.

[30] Roeser RW, Eccles JS, Sameroff AJ. School as a context of early adolescents' academic and social-emotional development: A summary of research findings. Elementary Sch J 2000;100(5):443-549.

[31] Chen X, Chen H, Kaspar V. Group social functioning and individual socioemotional and school adjustment in Chinese children. Merrill-Palmer Quart 2001;47(2):264-99.

[32] Wentzel KR. Family functioning and academic achievement in middle school: A social-emotional perspective. J Early Adolesc 1994;14(2):268-91.

[33] Dubow EF, Ippolito MF. Effects of poverty and quality of the home environment on changes in the academic and behavioural adjustment of elementary school-age children. J Clin Child Psychol 1994;23:401-12.
[34] Dubow EF, Arnett M, Smith K, Ippolito M. Predictors of future axpectations of inner-city children: A 9-month prospective study. J Early Adolesc 2001;21:5-28.
[35] Scott-Jones D. Parent-child interactions and school achievement. In: Ryan. BA, Adams. GR, Weissberg. RP, Hampton. RL, eds. The family-school connection. Thousand Oaks, CA: Sage, 1995:75-107.
[36] Simons-Morton BG, Crump AD. Association of parental involvement and social competence with school adjustment and engagement among sixth graders. J Sch Health 2003;73(3):121-6.
[37] Resnick MD, Harris LJ, Blum RW. The impact of caring and connectedness on adolescent health and well-being. J Pediatr Child Health 1993;29 (Suppl 1):S3-S9.
[38] Werner EE. Vulnerable but invincible: High risk children from birth to adulthood. Eur Child Adolesc Psychiatr 1996;5(Suppl 1):47-51.
[39] Wolin S, Wolin S. The resilient self: How survivors of troubled families rise above adversity. New York: Villard Books, 1993.
[40] Hetherington EM, Stanley-Hagan M. The adjustment of children with divorced parents: A risk and resiliency perspective. J Child Psychol Psychiatry 1999;40:129-40.
[41] World Health Organisation. Promoting health through schools. Report of a WHO expert committee on comprehensive school health education and promotion. Geneva: WHO Report Series 870, 1997.
[42] Poland BD, Green LW, Rootman I, eds. Settings for health promotion: Linking theory and practice. Thousand Oaks, CA: Sage, 2000.
[43] Markham WA, Aveyard P. A new theory of health promoting schools based on human functioning, school organisation and pedagogic practice. Soc Sci Med 2003;56:1209-20.
[44] Bronfenbrenner U. Ecological systems theory. Ann Child Dev 1989;6:187-249.
[45] King KA, Vidourek RA, Davis B, McClellan W. Increasing self-esteem and school connectedness through a multidimensional mentoring program. J Sch Health 2002;72(7):294-9.
[46] Lee A, Tsang C, Lee SH, To CY. A comprehensive "Healthy Schools Programme" to promote school health: The Hong Kong experience in joining the efforts of health and education sectors. J Epidemiol Commun Health 2003;57(3):174-82.
[47] Xu L, Pan B, Lin J, Chen L, Yu S, Jones J. Creating health-promoting schools in rural China: A project started from deworming. Health Promot Int 2000;15(3):197-206.
[48] Baker JA, Dilly LJ, Aupperlee JL, Patil SA. The developmental context of school satisfaction: School as psychologically healthy environment. Sch Psychol Quart 2003;18(2):206-21.
[49] Connell JP, Wellborn JG. Competence, automomy and relatedness: A motivational analysis of self-system processes. In: Gunnar M, Sroufe LA, eds. Minnesota Symposium of Child Psychology. Minneapolis, MN: University of Minnesota Press, 1991:43-77.

[50] Rutter M, Maughan B, Moretimore P, Ouston J, A. S. Fifteen thousand hours: Secondary schools and their effects on children. London: Open Books, 1979.
[51] Resnick M. Protecting adolescents from harm: Findings from the national longitudinal study on adolescent health. JAMA 1997;278(10):823-32.
[52] Hawkins J, Catalano R, Kosterman R, Abbot R, Hill K. Preventing adolescent health-risk behaviours by strengthening protection during childhood. Arch Paediatr Adolesc Med 1999;153(1):226-43.
[53] Nutbeam D, C. S, L. M, Bauman A. Warning! Schools can damage your health: Alienation from school and its impact on health behaviour. J Paediatrics Child Health 1993;29(1):S25-S30.
[54] Mortimore P, Sammons P, Stoll L, Lewis D, Ecob R. School matters: The junior years. Wells: Open Books, 1988.
[55] Hargreaves A, Earl L, Ryan J. Schooling for change: reinventing schools for early adolescents. London: Falmer, 1996.
[56] Catalano RF, Hawkins JD. The social development model: A theory of antisocial behaviour. In: Hawkins. JD, ed. Delinquency and crime: Current theories. New York: Cambridge University Press, 1996:149-97.
[57] Hawkins J, Catalano R, Miller J. Risk and protective factors for alcohol and other drug problems in adolescence and early adulthood: Implications for substance abuse prevention. Psychol Bull 1992;112(1):64-105.
[58] Hertzman C. Population health and human development. In: Keating DP, Hertzman C, eds. Developmental health and wealth of nations, social, biological and educational dynamics. New York: Guilford, 1999:21-40.
[59] Van der Gaag J. From child development to human development. In: Young ME, ed. From early child development to human development. Investing in our children's future. Washington, DC: World Bank, 2002:63-80.
[60] Vimpani G, Patton G, Hayes A. The relevance of child and adolescent development for outcomes in education, health and life success. Research Report. Melbourne: Australian Institute Family Studies, 2002.
[61] Shriver TP, Schwab-Stone M, DeFalco K. Why SEL is the better way: The New Haven Social Development Program. In: Cohen J, ed. Educating minds and hearts: Social emotional learning and the passage into adolescence. New York: Teachers College Press, 1999:43-60.
[62] Lanrieri L, Patti J. Waging peace in our schools. Boston: Beacon, 1996.
[63] Bronfenbrenner U. The ecology of human development: Experiments by nature and design. Cambridge: Harvard University Press, 1979.
[64] Sanders MG. The role of "community" in comprehensive school, family and community partnership programs. Elementary Sch J 2001;102(1):19-34.
[65] Gailmore R, Goldenberg C. Analysing cultural models and settings to connect minority achievement and school improvement research. Educ Psychol 2001;36(1):45-56.
[66] Taylor L, Adelman HS. Connecting schools, families and communities. Professional Sch Couns 2000;3(5):298-311.
[67] Sun J, Stewart D. How effective is the health promoting school approach in building social capital in primary schools? Health Educ 2007;107(6):556-74.

[68] McNeely C, Nonnemaker JM, Blum RW. Promoting school connectedness: Evidence from the national longitudinal study of adolescent health. J Sch Health 2002;72(4):138-47.

[69] Chen X, Chen H, Kaspar V, Noh S. Adolescent social, emotional and school adjustment in Mainland China. Int J Group Tensions 2000;29:51-78.

[70] Kinderman TA. Natural peer groups as contexts for individual development: The case of children's motivation in school. Dev Psychol 1993;29:970-7.

In: Health Promotion
Editors: J. Sun, N. Buys, J. Merrick
ISBN: 978-1-62257-870-2

Chapter II

Child abuse, neglect and maltreatment health service in Australia: A literature review

***Jing Sun, PhD*[*,1] *and Nicholas Buys, PhD*[2]**
[1]School of Public Health and Griffith Health Institute, Griffith University, Gold Coast Campus, Parkland, Gold Coast, Australia
[2]School of Human Services and Social Work, and Griffith Health Institute, Griffith University, Parkland, Gold Coast, Australia

Abstract

This chapter reviews child abuse, neglect and maltreatment health service practice in Australia. Child abuse, neglect and maltreatment and the need to protect children from harm and prevent abuse and neglect has become a significant public health concern. This chapter reviews current clinical and community practice in Australia in the following aspects: clinical governance, workforce development, early prevention and intervention, partnership, communication and coordination, and core activities development. It is recommended that the framework for child protection work should include the following: 1) Develop health service capacity

* *Correspondence:* Jing Sun, PhD, School of Public Health, Griffith University and Griffith Health Institute, Griffith University, Gold Coast Campus, Parkland, Q4222 Australia. E-mail: j.sun@griffith.edu.au.

with institution: Each health service district, hospital and departments need to develop service roles. 2) Develop district and department governance procedures. 3) Professional training provision. 4) Multi-disciplinary teamwork. 5) Develop personnel role and responsibilities package within each department 6) Stipulate clinical handover and care coordination procedures and 7) Develop early identification and early intervention strategies.

Introduction

Child abuse and neglect, and protection of children from the same, has become a significant clinical and community concern both in Australia and overseas (1-4). It is estimated that the prevalence of child physical abuse Australia ranges from 5-18% (5,6), prevalence of child neglect ranged from 2% to 12% (6,7).The prevalence estimates of child emotionally maltreated are quite different, ranging from 6% (8) to 17% (6); The prevalence of male child abuse was 1.4-8.0% for penetrative abuse and 5.7-16.0% for non-penetrative abuse, and prevalence rates female children was 4.0-12.0% for penetrative abuse and 13.9-36.0% for non-penetrative abuse (1-4). Given the significant impact of early experiences of violence, abuse and harsh parenting regimes on later development, it is important that children are protected effectively from potential harm.

Health services play a crucial role in recognising such harmful situations and taking immediate action to ensure the physical safety of children and minimize the long term emotional harm that accompanies abusive family, community, and social contexts. It is a common practice that Child Protection Health Services provide reporting and documentation to child protection service or child welfare services, assessing and diagnosing the children needing protection, investigating matters where a child is at possible risk of significant harm, and referral of children and families to social and health services that provide for the ongoing safety and well-being of the children. However, using an integrated approach to provide health services in child protection has not been evaluated. Physicians and nurses in many countries are legally required to refer suspicious child abuse or neglect cases to designated child welfare agencies. Reporting of child maltreatment is a challenging task (9,10), but protect children from harm becomes priority. Queensland Health, as a key stakeholder in the child protection work, has provided services in identification and reporting of suspected child abuse and neglect. To continue this role, a contemporary and effective service model to incorporate strategies and implementation plans in child protection is needed.

The aim of the Child Protection Service Delivery Project was to develop a comprehensive and effective health service model for a health district in Queensland Health. It is critical that this framework is evidence-based and informed by the best evidence and practices in child protection. This review of literature was undertaken in order to support the project team in service framework development and implementation.

Literature review

The main objective was to review the service delivery model in child protection in order to;

1. Inform and support the development of child protection service delivery framework in a Health Service District in Queensland.
2. Ensure the model is evidence-based and encompasses current best practice from other countries.

An extensive national and international literature search was conducted during June 2007-June 2008 using a variety of databases including academic databases [Medline from 1966 to December 2007, ProQuest from 1980 to 2007, Science Direct 1980 to 2007, Balckwell Syndergy from 1966 to 2007], Australian databases [Australian Institute of Family Studies Library Catalogue, Australian Public Affairs Information Service, Australian Family & Society Abstracts, CINCH (Australian Criminology Database), National clearinghouses in the fields of child protection, health and domestic violence], and international databases [Care Data, Child Abuse, Child Welfare and Adoption (NISC), Educational Resources Information Clearinghouse, National Criminal Justice Reference Service, Sociological Abstracts, Social Services Abstracts].

Search words for identifying the research on organizational risk factors, management, recruitment and assessment included child and worker, staff and child, exploitation and institutions, recruitment and child, actuarial and child, and actuarial and risk and assessment. For identification of research on child-related and perpetrator-related risk factors, the search words included child abuse and child abuser. The key words "child abuse", "physical", and "neglect" were used to search the literature. The results published before 1980 and in language other than English were used. Articles identified in the search were subdivided into Clinical governance, Workforce development, Early Prevention and Intervention, Partnership, Communication and coordination, Core activities, and Culturally and diverse background population. Articles with core activities were sought with the terms "case management" or "risk assessment". Additionally, the Child Abuse Quarterly Review of research on child maltreatment and the journal "Child Abuse and Neglect" from January 1995 to December 2007 were also reviewed.

Current knowledge and practices

No service framework at a district level was available either from literature review or from interstate. Therefore, the research team was required to determine relevant topics and issues to guide the selection and examination of the literature. After consultation with Child Protection Project team, the concept of Child Protection Service Delivery Framework was interpreted to have the following core dimensions:

1. Clinical governance
2. Workforce development
3. Early prevention and intervention
4. Partnership, communication and coordination
5. Core activities

Clinical governance

Clinical governance is the set of processes and systems that ensure the safety and highest quality of the process of care. It includes the systems for accountability, oversight and systematic improvement of care and a set of checks and reviews, whereby teams and communities of clinicians oversee and systematically improve the processes and practices of care (11). It was introduced in the 1990s in the National Health Service in the United Kingdom and has become popular in the UK, Canada and Australia (12).

Clinical governance is closely associated with functional health service units including the ward, unit, department, health centre and clinic. The governance of all units begins at the highest level, requiring the leadership to set up organisational agendas for corporate, district and clinical governance. Having adequate reporting mechanisms and reviewing clinical and organisational performance through accurate data on a regular basis are preconditions for effective leadership. Governing authorities need to ensure that the organisation is performing effectively, services are being delivered according to predefined standards, and mechanisms are in place to take remedial action when problems are encountered.

Describing the clinical governance framework for government, district and area service level in explicit terms is important for a number of reasons. First, it provides a clear and transparent communication of the organisation's intentions and expectations in relation to the delivery of care to all stakeholders. Second, it clarifies roles and responsibilities of consumers and staff across the organisation while explicitly demonstrating the value and contribution they bring to the service, and the interdependence of each person's roles and responsibilities. Third, it allows operationalization through the inclusion of relevant elements of the clinical governance framework in job descriptions, staff selection processes, performance review, education and training needs analysis, building of staff and service capacity, and testing and improvement of the framework's elements.

The Australian Council of Healthcare Standards (13), in 2004, defined clinical governance as *"the system by which the governing body, managers and clinicians share responsibility and are held accountable for patient safety, minimising risks to consumers and for continuously monitoring and improving the quality of care."* The application of clinical governance in a health care setting in Australia is new and the success of its implementation has not been evaluated. But a number of common principles have been proposed across Australia (14):

1. Collaborative relationship between clinicians and managers in which the specific roles and responsibilities of each are made explicit, are understood by the other and are complementary, and where the highly trained, skilled clinicians provide increasingly complex, evidenced-based care to high-risk patients in collaboration with managers who have the high level training and skills to manage and to change highly complex, high-risk health systems (15).
2. Safeguarding principles in clinical risk management, where doctors play a crucial role in protecting children from abuse and neglect (16). There is a legal and professional duty for all doctors to ensure that

advice provided, either to the child or young person or to their parents or carers, is appropriate and has taken into account any impact that this may have on the ultimate safety of the individual (16).

3. Strengthening the roles and responsibilities of clinicians in clinical governance, which has been identified as the mechanism to systematically improve standards of clinical care (17). Its components are evidence-based practice, audit, risk management, mechanisms to monitor the outcome of care, lifelong learning among clinicians, and systems for managing poor performance.
4. Monitoring and clinical supervision of nurses, the importance of which has been emphasized in past decade in a range of United Kingdom government and professional policy documents (17).
5. Maintaining effectiveness in clinical governance, where the medical audits were the first type of activity implemented in the National Health Service in United Kingdom. It is a process that strives to improve patient care and outcomes through systematic review of care against explicit criteria, the implementation of change at an individual, team, or service level, and further monitored to confirm improvement of service delivery. However, opinions about its effectiveness are mixed in United Kingdom(18), many seeing audit solely as an educational exercise for junior doctors and having a limited contribution due to lack of methodological rigour and the poor quality of resultant recommendations. Those with a more positive view saw national audits as especially useful, particularly when they had been developed with clinical input. Others highlighted the benefits of audits that were able to identify areas of clinical risk or explored a problem arising from a clinical incident in detail. Audit meetings were one mechanism for bringing together departments on different hospital sites, providing a building block for standardisation of services. Effective audits were seen as those that involved the whole team, including other health care professionals, and had consultant input into both the conduct of the audit and the implementation of the recommendations (18).
6. Facilitation of a more conducive cultural climate by the use of a variety of approaches, including reviewing and aligning policies, structures and processes within a clear vision and framework of goals related to quality improvement, reviewing and celebrating positive behaviours, involving staff in the process of change with support for any training and development needs, improving the effectiveness of

communication across the organization and providing teams with time and space to reflect upon their performance. All these have been shown to have a positive effect (19-21).

Clinical governance includes systems for accountability, oversight and systematic improvement of care (15), where the use of sound evidence as a basis for management of decision-making is been increasingly acknowledged. A vital focus in effective application of clinical governance principles to the development of enhanced systems of performance management for nursing, medical and technical staff, including staff appraisal and ensuring continued professional development (15). Clinical governance has been found critical to the successful development and implementation of an effective "system" approach to patient safety in health care (22). Developing clinical governance at corporate level rests on the core processes of clinical audit, clinical effectiveness, clinical risk management (CRM), quality assurance, and organisational and staff development. CRM is a key driver of patient safety processes within a clinical governance structure. There is a variation observed in the knowledge, beliefs and attitudes of experienced staff concerning clinical governance and CRM processes because;

- The clinical governance and CRM processes currently being operationalised in the Australian health care sector are relatively new in Australia;
- There is a lack of attention to these issues in the Australian child protection literature;
- There is a lack of educational opportunities at both undergraduate and post registration levels for nurses to develop knowledge and skills relevant to clinical governance and CRM;
- The predictable resistance of a minority of staff to change (12,23).

Workforce development

Health care workers, ranging from clinical staff who are responsible for conducting specialist medical investigations, to nurses working the community in positions such as school nurses, midwives and health visitors, have been recognised as having a key role in the child protection service internationally and in Australia. While child abuse work may constitute one of many responsibilities, nurses and paediatricians are often the first professionals to identify children who have been or are at significant risk of child abuse and neglect. However, the potential for nurses and paediatricians to fulfil this role in many settings is hampered by a perceived lack of training around child protection (24). Most studies show that the training for child protection workforce is inadequate in many countries, and has highlighted the need for adequate for initial and continued training in the identification, assessment and intervention in child protection, for all health professionals in primary and tertiary health care in regular contact with children,(25-27).

The findings from inquiries and research suggest that in order to provide an effective child protection service, primary care workers need both the skills and knowledge to identify cases of child abuse and to know their roles and responsibilities, as well as how to liaise with other agencies involved in child protection. Fifty eight percent of services in United Kingdom did not have enough trained nurses (28). It is particularly important that front line nurses are well trained so that they can draw the attention of designated child protection staff to any cases of concern. Seventy percent of services nationally did not have enough trained nurses at this level. Eight-five percent of services in Accident and Emergency departments did not meet the standard training in child protection service (29). In the United Kingdom, with identification of training needs of already qualified nurses in the field of child protection (30, 31), it has been suggested that mandatory qualifying and in-service training should be provided to enable nurses to identify, assess and refer children for protection. The Royal College of Nursing (28) has produced guidelines with regard to the extent and level of training required by nurses in child protection.

Further, given the rising scale of expectations placed on general medical practitioners (GPs) in taking on responsibility for child protection, it is essential to provide them with the skill, knowledge, attitudes, and values in this area of practice. However, a survey conducted in Canada found that among 16 medical schools, only 3 programs had mandatory clinical training for residents, and nine programs offered electives in child protection which were taken during the previous year by only 4.7% of respondents (32). Overall, only 26.8% of the residents have had any kind of clinical instruction in child protection at any time during their medical training. Over 91% of residents and 85% of fourth-year residents have indicated their need of further training in this area.

Within Australia and New Zealand, advanced training in child protection workforce falls within the scope of Community Child Health. Recently, advanced trainees who work under the Specialist Advisory Committee for

Community Child Health are required to complete 3 months of training in child protection. The child protection paediatrician may participate in multidisciplinary meetings, and participate in shared decision-making. In their clinical work, they may be called upon to advocate for the child for services and assess the development and behaviour of children who may have experienced abuse or neglect (9,33). One-third of CP paediatricians have reported receiving no training at all in child protection, and two thirds of CP paediatricians have received less than 4 months of training prior to completing their FRACP. Those paediatricians contribute to decision making with other child protection stake-holders in multi-agency meetings, and 50% of paediatricians indicated that they had less than adequate training for this role prior to FRACP (9, 33).Most paediatricians spend half of their allocated child protection time assessing children referred to the child protection system from health services. Only 13% of their working week is spent on the ongoing medical follow up of these children. In addition, only 50% of paediatrician continue to manage behavioural or developmental problems identified in these children beyond 6 months (9) suggesting that half these high-risk children receive long-term management elsewhere. Doctors who take on such tasks need additional opportunities for training and professional development, and a means of accreditation that confirms their expertise to clinical and forensic colleagues and to the judiciary.

Nurses in Australia, who have considerable contacts with children, such as midwives, school nurses and nurses in paediatric wards or acute hospitals did not provide services in child protection, reflecting the fact that these services are provided by other departments (24). The challenge to provide adequate training to nurses who have identified a need for further knowledge about child protection issues is great, especially given a lack of consensus among most groups of nurses as to what training they require.

Early prevention and early intervention

The early identification of child maltreatment and early intervention to reduce the degree of harm in children is critical to child's physical and psychological development (29). The main strategies in early identification and intervention discussed in the literature are identification of children and parents who fall into high risk groups and identification of risk factors.

Child maltreatment is usually the result of interaction of many risk factors, such as presence of a disability (34), a parent with substance abuse and/or depression (35), intimate partner violence within the family (36), residence in dangerous neighbourhoods or poor recreational facilities, and poverty and associated burdens (37). The family, community and the health department are collectively responsible for the children's safety within their families. When the child maltreatment occurs and an adult fails his/her role to protect a child from harm, child protection system becomes responsible to provide service response by providing primary, secondary and tertiary services.

The goal of primary health services is to provide support and education for children and families before problems arise. In many cases, primary services prevent abuse and neglect occurring, are offered to everyone, and include ante-natal services, maternal and child health services and human relationship education in schools.

Community education and awareness programs focus on addressing community attitudes towards violence, children's rights and physical punishment which are associated with child abuse. These programs educate the public about alternatives to abuse, changing social attitudes towards violence, and encourage community debate about issues such as censorship, family violence, substance abuse and drug use, etc. Physicians can help prevent child maltreatment in several ways (38). Establishing a good relationship with a family provide opportunities to observe parent-child relationship and identify risk of potential harm from adults.

In many countries, all new births are notified to the nurses and they have a minimum of five contacts during the first year of life which take place at prescribed times, although in practice there may be more frequent visits if necessary (39). School- aged children are followed up through the school nursing service, which plays an important role in child protection due to the routine contact with all young children and their families (40). For example, in Ireland, a breakdown of time spent on domiciliary child development visits shows that 82% of time is given over to developmental checks, 1.5% to ante-natal care, 14.7% to visiting vulnerable families and 2.1% to family surveillance (41).

Parental education is useful to help with diminishing the risk of child abut and maltreatment. Hospital based programs can be developed to educate parents about infants behaviours and the parental methods to prevent abusive physical injury. Health check-up can provide opportunities to check psychosocial risks, such as parental depression, substance use, domestic violence, financial strains and stresses. However, the primary care role of advising and supporting parents to prevent poor child health care practices and child maltreatment has not yet been evaluated. Gough (42) in an extensive review of the literature on child abuse interventions suggests that interventions such as education and support may not be evaluated because of the difficulties inherent in measurement of their effectiveness.

Nurses can refer to statutory and voluntary agencies before any problems arise and they may play an effective role in primary protection of children (43). The Dublin-based Community Mothers' Programme provides an example of how nurses' work effectively through the identification of community needs, and initiation and referral of children and families to support programmes (43).

There are several types of service provision for child protection at a primary health care level (44):

- Universal (core) health visiting: The new birth visit was the cornerstone of the universal health visiting service, which predicted more postnatal home visits and more frequent group and community-based activities.
- Teamwork delivering core service: The core service was delivered, in most instances, by the health visitor in conjunction with others, including members of the wider primary care team. Where health visitors led a skill-mix team, fewer scheduled home visits occurred, but there were more group and community activities overall.
- Extra health visiting: Services included additional home visits by health visitors and by other team members for service provision with regard to postnatal depression, breast-feeding, parenting education, sleep or behaviour problems, domestic violence, drug users and support, menopause, weight management, men's health, language support, speech and language development, learning difficulties, mental health, multiple births, rural health and sexual health.

Secondary prevention is concerned with the early identification and appropriate referral of families once there is evidence of risk of child abuse and neglect. Secondary health services include in-home family support, counselling, respite care and various parenting and self-help groups. The secondary role of the nurses and paediatricians in early detection of families at risk is grounded in their expertise of normal emotional and physical development of children in the context of their families, as well as in an in-depth knowledge and awareness of injuries or behaviour likely to be non-accidental in nature (45).

Currently, reporting a child on an "at risk" is mandatory in Australia (45,46). In the presence of an 'at risk' reporting, there is a formal mechanism for differentiating between 'vulnerable' and 'at-risk' children. Consequently, a family may be protected from the situation as 'vulnerable' and/or 'at risk'. However, in many Western Countries, the need to differentiate these criteria remains largely unarticulated. This has led to nurses and paediatricians retaining responsibility for child protection in situations where specialist intervention is required.

Tertiary prevention deals with minimizing disabilities. Greenwalt, Sklare, and Portes (47) described the current practice of some mental health practitioners in the treatment of cases involving physical child abuse in America. The family is considered the primary client most frequently with the focus of the family therapy to stop the abuse and to improve family relationships. Whether this focus should be considered the primary therapeutic goal needs further longitudinal research on the abused child.

One would expect physically abused children to receive the help needed to stabilize their lives and become productive members of society as soon as possible. However, while some authorities recognize the importance of providing treatment for the abused child (48), little can be found in the literature about the treatment actually provided to the victim (49). White (50) notes mental health services to the abused child only as a part of foster care, residential care, or day care but not in the context of health service. Greater emphasis appears to be placed on the treatment of the parents and the safety of the child (51) than on overcoming the effects of the abuse on the child.

Partnership, communication and coordination

Interagency coordination and collaboration is a significant issue for the provision of child protection and family support services. A coordinated response to the problem of child maltreatment can produce more effective risk assessment, greater efficiency in the use of resources, improved service delivery by the avoidance of duplication and overlap between existing services, clarification of agency or professional roles and responsibilities in front-line problems and demarcation disputes, and the delivery of comprehensive services.

The structures or mechanisms that facilitate interagency collaboration and coordination are referral protocols, case conferencing, and the development of multidisciplinary teams. The formal referral protocols between health departments and social workers are mostly the primary means of communication. Informal linkages in conjunction with formal communication structures appears to be an effective partnership and coordination between agencies (52). The collaboration between medical evaluation for abused children and local child protection social (CPS) workers is needed, and to achieve agreement between paediatricians and CP workers are critical to identify the cases and improve the services (53).

Standardising decision making, information sharing, consensus decision making, mediation by an administrator in the absence of consensus, rational discussions among members of the team and supportive attitudes towards other members, leading role played by the persons with most first-hand knowledge about the case handled, and the decisions made are respected despite the status of the person in team, all lead to better service provision (54). In Queensland, where child protection and adult mental health are the responsibility of separate government departments-the Department of Communities and Queensland Health, workers engage in collaboration to provide a wide range of services and supports focusing on adult mental health, child protection, family counselling and support, child health and mental health, and legal and financial assistance (55). The provision of these various supports is delivered via a highly fragmented and decentralised network of over 100 government (federal, state and local) and community-based programs, services and agencies.

In some respects, the respondents' description of their experiences of interagency collaboration was encouraging. In half the cases reported, respondents identified that either no issues had arisen, or that collaboration had resulted in an improved outcome for the client or a positive collaborative process for the workers. This finding supports previous research, indicating that collaboration can be rewarding and beneficial for both workers and clients. However, in one-third of cases communication was cited as a problem and support previous findings (56-58) which indicate that information sharing, communication, and negotiating issues of confidentiality are crucial to a successful collaborative relationship. The second most commonly cited difficulty was the need for role clarity, including boundaries and leadership. This result supports the findings of Mizrahi and Rosenthal (59), which found leadership to be the most important factor for successful coalitions. This raises the questions of who the leader should be, how leaders should be chosen, and the scope of the authority to be bestowed.

It is evident that effective communication and collaboration between health professionals on child protection issues is related to organisational level strategies, case level strategies, inter-professional relationships, staff training and supervision, types of knowledge required, and understanding of the interdependent needs of parents and children (55). Policy and practice is closely linked to effective partnerships. With high incidents of child maltreatment in Queensland (60), the state department of health, hospital-based child protection teams, nurses, and medical practitioners are increasingly asked to evaluate and treat child abuse and neglect despite their lack of formal training. In an effort to manage increased caseloads, other disciplines have trained paraprofessionals and lay people such as parent aides, lay therapists, and lay health visitors to provide services to abusive families. These workers have been shown to be fully capable of identifying abusive situations, and have alleviated workloads and provided additional services.

In Australia, Departments of Health (DOH) plays a coordinating role in addressing child abuse and domestic violence through developing Mental Health Policy and Framework, and establishing partnerships with other agencies and service uses. The partnership was particularly in areas such as multi-professional training, service delivery, continuation of health and social services for families, and referrals. One way of achieving closer cooperation among the various agencies involved in child protection work is through the establishment of 'multidisciplinary' or interagency teams or meetings (61). Most of the literature emphasizes the efficiency of this multidisciplinary approach to case consultation and its positive effect on service delivery (61).

There are several guides to the development and implementation of a multidisciplinary child protection team. One model is case consultation teams. These teams focus on case conferences, service development, and work to enhance interagency collaborations (61). Another model is treatment teams, often in hospitals, which collaborate on treatment plans for abused children and their families. They may also provide some long-term case management (62). A third model is resource development teams. These address the issue of child maltreatment through public education and advocacy. Members may be professionals working in the field or other citizens (63). Their program strengthens natural support networks through self-help groups and skills training sessions. The literature also describes mixed model teams that combine the above functions.

Child maltreatment in all its manifestations constitutes a diagnostic and therapeutic problem to all hospital personnel caring for children and adolescents. To optimise practical procedures and to ensure child protection independent of decisions made by any single person, several Austrian hospitals have formed child protection teams or child abuse and neglect teams. In 1999, the Federal Ministry for the Environment, Youth and Family published a recommendation to install Child Protection Team (CPT) in all paediatric departments in Austria and provided a set of guidelines to assist CPT in carrying out their work in paediatric hospitals. These guidelines currently form the constitutional basis of CPT in 68% of all Austrian paediatric hospitals. The CPT team comprises the following professionals groups: paediatricians, paediatric surgeons, a child and adolescent psychiatrics, psychologists, psychotherapists, nurses, a social worker and a secretary. The CPT is available only to inpatient and was founded principally as a tool to provide support to the staff on the individual wards of the departments involved. Inpatient data from CPT functioning in hospitals are relatively scarce in the literature. The detailed data about the functioning and effectiveness of CPT are available only from the USA and Canada. Unfortunately, in its current form the function of CPTs lacks a suitable quality assurance structure (both qualitative and financial-structural), as has also been documented in US CPTs. An improvement in this could ensure a better detection of maltreatment, a more appropriate handling of the whole problem and guaranteed protection of the children concerned.

Core activities

Nurses and paediatrician are often the first contact of children who are abused and neglected, and their education provides them with a broad base in assessment, planning, implementing and evaluating health care and nursing care in holistic way. They are responsible for primary, secondary and tertiary level of protection. The bulk of the responsibility in identifying and managing child maltreatment therefore lies with the health care teams.

There are many indicators that could help health professionals to identify the children at risk of maltreatment. These include inconsistent history, delay in seeking attention, parent-child interaction, and mismatch in history and examination. However, there has been a lack of clarity about the purpose and appropriate use of indicators of concern. For example, in Emergency department (ED), ED physicians limited their documentation to a single presenting complaint, and it was difficult to be certain that a particular indicator was looked for and not found (e.g, whether the child had an unclothed examination or only the symptomatic limb was examined). The documentation of childhood injuries in the ED is inadequate, making any assessment of abuse difficult. On review of the medical record, there was high percentage of children who had one or more indicators that merited further analysis before a diagnosis of accident could be assigned. However, only 0.9% of children were referred to further examination. The poor referral rate in ED suggests that ED and orthopaedic staff are unaware of the significance of the indicators of maltreatment.

In a study conducted in United Kingdom (64), it has been found that a large number of the protocols in ED department included long lists of signs and symptoms of abuse with no guidance on how to use these. Those with practical value included a short checklist, with clear guidelines on what to do if concerns were identified. Some indicators were very specific (for example, children under 1 year with a fracture, burn or scale), while others were more descriptive (for example, the parents behaviour gives rise to concern). One included recognised risk factors (for example, teenage parents, low income, or prematurity) as well as signs and symptoms, but gave no indicator on how these were to be interpreted.

Tertiary protection in the Australian and New Zealand context consists of medical follow-up for children entering the child protection system, and monitoring of the development and behavioural progress in these children beyond 6 months, involvement of preventative child protection programmes which include programs on high-risk families with young infants and child protection research (65). Most paediatricians who are doing tertiary protection may also get involved in the advocacy for the child for services through joining in multidisciplinary meetings, and participate with other child protection agency stake-holders in decisions aimed to achieve the best child protection outcomes (65).

The management of maltreated children has a number of options. For both sexual and physical abuse, cognitive-behavioural therapy (CBT) has dominated as the treatment with the most empirical validation. Parent training, in which parents are taught how to behaviourally specify goals for change, to track target behaviours, to positively reinforce pro-social conduct, and to punish or ignore their children's aversive behaviours have also been extended to include coping skills, self-control skills, communication skills training and psycho-education (66). Some interventions have been developed specifically for children who have been physically abused. These include peer training, a school-based intervention that uses pro-social peers to help children who are withdrawn to develop social skills (67). For children up to five years of age, a therapeutic child development program has been developed to provide an intensive milieu of services, such as nutrition, health care, developmental therapies, and case management, provided by responsive adults (68).

Group treatment has been a typical modality of intervention for sexual abuse given its cost effectiveness and potential to reduce stigma. The theoretical orientations of group therapy have varied widely and include most commonly eclectic treatment models comprising various combinations of the following components: psycho-education regarding sexual abuse and sexual abuse prevention, exploration of the abuse experience, exploration of feelings, art therapy, play therapy, role plays, problem solving, puppet work, writing exercises, and behaviour management (69, p.674).

Service delivery model for child protection

Based on the evidence from the literature review it is recommended that every health district and hospital have formal surveillance and accountability procedures or a clinical governance framework to improve quality and safety. To succeed, these frameworks must: 1) devolve governance and performance monitoring to the level of clinical units or departments where care is provided and whose staff bears the ultimate responsibility; 2) feature practice-relevant, data-driven agendas that actively seek involvement and innovation on the part of practising clinicians, and; 3) require hospital executives, clinical governance units and quality improvement coordinators to sponsor and support quality and safety activities within units. A relevant action plan should be developed for improving quality and safety and implement the clinical governance framework incorporating work force development and early identification and intervention into the implementation plan (70). This plan may include;

- Develop service delivery capacity: health service districts, hospitals and its departments should develop delivery capacity in relation to facilities, staffing, and management.

- Develop district and department governance procedures: The governance structure and procedure should be developed from state government executive to district and health area managers' level. This procedure should inform practice based framework and be implemented to the hospitals and districts.
- Professional training provision in child safety: Health department, universities, specialty collages, and medical societies should collaborate in forging new training programmes and career paths that focus on optimizing quality and safety. A key reform is to enable doctors, nurses and allied health professionals to more effectively undertake high-order bedside tasks that require specialised training by devolving and distracting, low-order clerical and non-clinical procedural tasks to appropriately trained assistants. In times of future shortages of specific groups of skilled clinicians, professional boundaries will need some renegotiation in situations where evidence confirms that tasks previously considered as the exclusive province of one type of practitioner can be safely carried out by other groups.
- Develop multi-disciplinary teamwork: Interdisciplinary team activities should be developed to reduce the risk of harm of children. Education and training should be provided to train multi-discipliny team's safety procedures, team skills and communication skills.
- Establish clinical orientation procedures: All hospital departments should provide all newly appointed clinicians and nurses with a multidisciplinary orientation and information package that outlines departmental policies and procedures and personnel roles and responsibilities.
- Develop clinical care coordination procedures: All hospital departments should have clear procedures for (1) clinical handover between shifts for all disciplines and between different care teams, (2) accessing information and advice from external caregivers (e.g., general practitioner and specialists) with regards to the suspicion of children who are abused and neglected, (3) recording clinical information arising from emergency and paediatric department clinics, case conference and consultant visits and conveying it to others who need to know, and (4) transferring structured child information (clinic identification and assessment and community referrals) to general practitioners and other clinicians involved in the clinical care.

- Implement early identification and early intervention practices: The health system is often the only infrastructure that reaches children younger than three years and therefore can initiate programmes to promote early development and prevent risks. In new born infant health check and health visits program, early detection of child abuse and neglect should be one of paediatricians' and nurses' tasks. Once children are identified to be at risk of potential harm referrals to relevant early intervention program should be made. The parenting program (e.g., Triple P parenting program) should be made available in clinical and community settings. The educational system can promote child development by supporting comprehensive programmes for early child development. If the programmes are of high quality, have family involvement, and when needed provide health care and food supplementation or micronutrients, evidence suggests that disparities among the most disadvantaged children can be reduced before school entry. Linking early development programmes administered through the health system with programmes in the educational system increases the likelihood of building intervention follow-up for children at risk. To increase coverage of early child development programmes and improve their quality and effectiveness, better advocacy strategies, coordination mechanisms, and improved policy are needed. Research is required on approaches to delivering feasible effective child protection programmes at scale and on the effects of synergies on child outcomes.
- Implement pre and in-service training for health professionals development: Training local frontline health and social services professionals, and providing support and consultation in child protection is needed. Health professionals who were trained with knowledge and skills increase the rate of detection of child abuse and neglect (70). Due to the key role that nurses have in protecting children, specialist training in child protection needs to be provided to all nurses including those who do not work directly with children. They need to be able to access information on child protection issues as required. Many nurses work either directly with children or indirectly in settings where children may be present (e.g., in private homes or in clinics where children accompany parents who are service users). This includes district nurses, community psychiatric nurses, and nurses working in the fields of learning disability and addiction. If they are to effectively contribute to the child protection

agenda, they need at least some basic training about child protection, particularly around identifying children at risk and responding to any cases of suspected or alleged abuse of children. For new staff, participation in such training could be incorporated into their induction program, especially if an on-line training package is developed to provide basic knowledge about child protection issues.

References

[1] Dunne MP, Purdie DM, Cook MD, Boyle FM, Najman JM. Is child sexual abuse declining? Evidence from a population-based survey of men and women in Australia. Child Abuse Negl 2003;27(2):141-52.

[2] Mazza D, Dennerstein L, Garamszegi CV, Dudley EC. The physical, sexual and emotional violence history of middle-aged women: a community-based prevalence study. Med J Aust 2001;175(4):199-201.

[3] Moore EE, Romaniuk H, Olsson CA, Jayasinghe Y, Carlin JB, Patton GC. The prevalence of childhood sexual abuse and adolescent unwanted sexual contact among boys and girls living in Victoria, Australia. Child Abuse Negl 2010;34(5):7-.

[4] Najman JM, Dunne MP, Purdie DM, Boyle FM, Coxeter PD. Sexual abuse in childhood and sexual dysfunction in adulthood: an Australian population-based study. Arch Sex Behav 2005;34(5):517-26.

[5] Cohen RA, Paul RH, Stroud L, Gunstad J, Hitsman BL, McCaffery J, et al. Early life stress and adult emotional experience: an international perspective. Int J Psychiatr Med 2006;36(1):35-52.

[6] Price-Robertson R, Smart D, Bromfield L. Family is for life: How childhood experiences within the family help or hinder the lives of young adults. Fam Matters 2010;85:7-17.

[7] Straus MA, Savage SA. Neglectful behavior by parents in the life history of university students in 17 countries and its relation to violence against dating partners. Child Maltreat 2005;10(2):124-35.

[8] Rosenman S, Rodgers B. Childhood adversity in an Australian population. Soc Psychiatry Psychiatr Epidemiol 2004;39(9):695-702.

[9] Commission for Children and Young People and Child. Commission for Children and Young People and ChildGuardian Act 2000. Brisbane: Commission for Children and Young People and Child, 2001 Reprinted as in force on 1 July 2008. Report No.

[10] Flaherty EG, Sege R. Barriers to physician identification and reporting of child abuse. Pediatr Annu 2005;34:349-56.

[11] Gunn VL, Hickson GB, Cooper WO. Factors affecting pediatricians' reporting of suspected child maltreatment. Ambulent Pediatr 2005;5(96-101).

[12] Hoyle P. The promise of clinical governance. Royal Australasian College of Medical Administrator, 2006.

[13] Braithwaite J, Travaglia JF. An overview of clinical governance policies, paractices and initiatives. Aus Health Rev2008;32(1).
[14] Australian Council of Health Care Standards (ACHS). National report on health services accreditation performance. Accessed 2013 Mar 10. URL: www.achs.org.au.
[15] Scott IA, Poole PJ, Jayathissa S. Improving quality and safety of hospital care: a reappraisal and an agenda for clinically relevant reform. Int Med J 2008;38:44-55.
[16] O'Conner N, Paton M. Governance of and governance by: implementing a clinical governance framework in an area mental health service. Australasian Psychiatr 2008;16(2):69-73.
[17] Cowan J. Children and young people: reviewing practice and policies. Clin Governance Int J 2008;13(1):73-8.
[18] Department of Health. The nursing, midwifery and health visiting contribution to health and health care. London: Department Health, 1993.
[19] Hogan H, Basnett I, McKee M. Consultant's attitudes to clinical governance: Barriers and incentives to engagement. Public Health 2007;121:614-22.
[20] Blumenthal D, Kilo C. A report card on continuous quality-improvement. Milbank Q 1998;76(625-648).
[21] Locock L. Redesigning health care: New wine from old bottles. J Health Service Res Policy. 2003;8:120-2.
[22] Morrison P, Heineke J. Why do health practitioners resist quality management. Quality Progress 1992;25:51-5.
[23] Johnstone M, Kanitsaki O. Patient safety and the integration of graduate nurses into effective organisational clinical risk management systems and processes: An Australian study. Organizational Manage Health Care 2008;17(2):162-73.
[24] Swerissen H, Jordan L. Clinical governance in community health care settings: Evidence and issues. Aust J Primary Health 2005;11(2):26-31.
[25] Crisp BR, Lister PG. Nurses' perceived training needs in chldr protection issues. Health Educ 2006;106(5):381-99.
[26] Laming L. The Victoria Climbie Inquiry: Report of an inquiry by Lord Laming. London: HMSO, 2003.
[27] Hammond H. Child protection inquiry into the circumstances surrounding the death of Kennedy McFarlane. Edinburgh: Dumfries Galloway Child Protection Committee, 2001.
[28] Lupton C, Khan P, North N, Lacy D. The role of health professionals in the Child Protection process. Portsmouth: Social Services Research Unit, University Portsmouth, 2000 21.
[29] Royal College of Nursing. Child protection. Every nurse's responsibility. London: RCN, 2003.
[30] Quin G, Evans R. Accident and emergency department access to the child protection register: a questionnaire survey. EMJ 2002;19:136-7.
[31] Powell C. Child protection: The crucial role of hte children's nurse. Paediatr Nurs 1997;9(9):13-6.
[32] Thoebald S. Child protection. Why continuing education for nurses is important. Pediatr Nurs 2000;12(3):6-7.
[33] Murray T. Child protection neglected in pediatric training. Med Post 2002;38(25):1.

[34] Gunn VL, Hickson GB, Cooper WO. Factors affecting pediatricians' reporting of suspected child maltreatment. Ambulent Pediatr 2005;5:96-101.

[35] Kendall-Tackett K, Lyon T, Taliaferrro G, Little L. Why child maltreatment researchers should include children's disability status in their maltreatment studies. Child Abuse Negl 2005;29:147-51.

[36] Wilson SL, Kuebli JE, Hughes HM. Patterns of maternal behavior among neglectful families: implications for research and intervention. Child Abuse Negl 2005;29:985-1001.

[37] Korbin JE. Neighborhood and community connectedness in child maltreatment research. Child Abuse Negl 2003;27:137-40.

[38] Sedlack AJ, Bdroadhurst DD. Third national incidece study of child abuse and neglect: final report. Washington, DC: US Department Health Human Services, 1996.

[39] Dubowitz H. Preventing child gengecta nd physical abuse: A role for pediatricians. Pediatr Rev 2002;23:191-6.

[40] Kelly A. A public health nursing perspective. In: Fergusson H, Kenny P, eds. Behalf of the child: Child welfare, child protection and the Child Care Act 1991. Bublin: AA Farmar, 1995:186-202.

[41] Gilligan R. Irish child care services-Policy, practice and provision. Dublin: Institute Public Administration, 1991.

[42] Burke TP. Survey of the workload of public health nurses. Dublin, Ireland: Institute Community Health Nursing, 1986.

[43] NSW Department of Health. Child Protection Service Plan 2004-2007. In: Health NDo, editor: NSW Department of Health 2004; 2004.

[44] Queensland Health. Strategic Policy Framework for Children's and Young People's Health 2002-2007. Brisbane, QLD: Queensland Health, 2002.

[45] Gough D, Bell M. Providing services for children and young People who have experienced sexual abuse. Child Abuse Rev 2005;14:1-3

[46] Johnson Z, Howell F, Molloy B. Community mothers programme: randomised contorlled trial of non-professional interveniton in parenting. BMJ 1993;306:1449-52.

[47] Cowley S, J. BR. Resources revisited: salutogenesis from a lay perspective. J Adv Nurs 1999;29:994-1004.

[48] Greenwalt BC, Sklare G, Portes P. The therapeutic treatment provided in cases involving physical child abuse: A description of current practices. Child Abuse Negl 1998;22(1):71-8.

[49] Choy S. The psychological perspective. In: Untalan FF, Mills CS, eds. Interdisciplinary perspectives in child abuse and neglect. New York: Praeger, 1992.

[50] Graziano AM, Mills JR. Treatment for abused children: When is a partial solution acceptable? Child Abuse Negl 1992;16:217-28.

[51] White JC. The role of the social worker. In: Bross DC, Michaels LF, eds. Foundations of child advocacy: Legal representation of the maltreated child. Longmont, CO: Bookmakers Guild, 1987:61-70.

[52] Elmer E, Schultz BS. Social work evaluation and family assessment. In: D.C. Bross DC, Krugman RD, Lenherr MR, Rosenberg DA, Schmitt BD, ed. The new child protection team handbook. New York: Garland, 1988:136-49.

[53] Tomison AM, ed. Interagency collaboration and communication in child protection cases: some findings from an Australian case tracking study. Paper presented at the Fifth ISPCAN Asian Conference on Child Protection; 26-28 November, 1999; Hong Kong: National Child Protection Clearing House, Australian Institute of Family Studies.

[54] Campbell KA, Bogen DL, Berger RP. The other children. A survey of child abuse physicians on the medical evaluation of children living with a physically abused child. Arch Pediatr Adolesc Med 2006;160:1241-6.

[55] Tomison A, Poole L. Preventing child abuse and neglect: Findings from an Australian audit of prevention programs. Melbourne, Australia: Australian Institute Family Studies, 2000.

[56] Darlington Y, Feeney JA. Collaboration between mental health and child protection services: Professionals' perceptions of best practice. Child Youth Serv Rev 2008;30(2):187-98.

[57] Bailey S. Confidentiality and young people: Myths and realities. In: Cordess C, editor. Confidentiality and mental health. London: Jessica Kingsley, 2001:71-84.

[58] Morrison T. Partnership and collaboration: Rhetoric and reality. Child Abuse Negl 1996;20(2):127-40.

[59] Pietsch J, Short L. Working together: Families in which a parent has a mental illness: Developing 'best practice' for service provision and interagency collaboration. Melbourne, Australia: Mental Health Research Institute, 1998.

[60] Mizrahi T, Rosenthal BB. Complexities of coalition building: Leaders' successes, strategies, struggles, and solutions. Social Work 2001;46(1):63-78.

[61] Crocker D. Innovative models for rural child protection teams. Child Abuse Negl 1996;20(3):205-11

[62] Gentry T, Brisbane FL. The solution for child abuse rests with the community. Children Today 1982:22-4.

[63] Miller JL, Whittaker JK. Social services and social support: blended programs for families at risk of child maltreatment. Child Welfare 1988;67.(2):161-74.

[64] Sidebotham P, Biu T, Goldsworthy L. Child protection procedures in emergency departments. Emergency Med J 2008;24:831-5.

[65] Cruickshanks P, Skellern C. Role of the tertiary child protection paediatrician: Expert and advocate. J Paediatr Child Health 2007;43:34-9.

[66] Kolko DJ. Clinical monitoring of treatment course in child physical abuse: psychometric characteristics and treatment comparisons. Child Abuse Negl1996;20:23-43.

[67] Fantuzzo JW, Wray L, Hall R, Goins C, Azar S. Parent and social-skills training for mentally retarded mothers identified as child maltreaters. Am J Mental Defic 1986;91:135-40.

[68] Moore E, Seattle WA, Armsden G, Seattle W, Gogerty PL. A twelve-year follow-up study of maltreated and at-risk children who received early therapeutic child care. Child Maltreat 1998;3(1):3-16.

[69] Deare JR. A meta-analytic investigation of group treatment outcomes for sexually abused children. Child Abuse Negl 1997;21(7):669-80.
[70] Cerezo MA, Pons-Salvador G. Improving child maltreatment detection systems: a large-scale case study involving health, social services, and school professionals. Child Abuse Negl 2004;28(11):1153-69.

In: Health Promotion
Editors: J. Sun, N. Buys, J. Merrick
ISBN: 978-1-62257-870-2

Chapter III

Managing Occupational Stress Injury in Police Services: A Literature Review

Christine Randall, PhD[1] and Nicholas Buys, PhD[1,2]*
[1]School of Human Services and Social Work, Griffith University, Parkland, Gold Coast, Australia
[2]Griffith Health Institute, Griffith University, Parkland, Gold Coast, Australia

Abstract

Occupational stress is an increasingly significant economic and social burden in Australia, yet its impact is not being adequately addressed, particularly in emergency services organisations, such as police services. Management of workplace stress injury is therefore a priority, requiring integration of effective occupational rehabilitation systems to prevent and mitigate this condition at an organisational level. This literature review describes the specific issues associated with occupational stress in police services. Findings of the review indicate that attention is required to the job and organisational characteristics of police services, stress

* *Correspondence:* Professor Nicholas Buys, PhD, School of Human Services and Social Work, Griffith University, Australia. E-mail: n.buys@griffith.edu.au

management processes, training and knowledge, and the police culture and organisational climate. These issues contribute to stress and create barriers to rehabilitation within police services. Recommendations for addressing occupational stress in police organisations are provided, with a focus on developing and maintaining effective prevention and rehabilitation processes.

Introduction

Stress in the work context is a significant issue given the economic impact on employers and society. The median cost for a mental disorders claim in Australia was calculated at $18,000 in 2008-09, whilst the median cost for all serious workers' compensation claims during the same period was $7,700 (1). There are considerable indirect and hidden costs associated with stress injury (2). For example, workplace stress significantly affects employee productivity, absenteeism and presenteeism, with an estimated overall cost of over $10 billion per year (2-4). Hidden costs are also associated with staff turnover, the impact of stress on physical health, such as cardiovascular disease and musculoskeletal disorders, and the consequences for families and society. The direct and indirect costs of stress suggest that employers need to manage this condition in the workplace to ensure their businesses remain competitive.

In Australia, employers have a legal obligation to prevent and manage workplace injuries. This includes the provision of safe work environments, workers' compensation insurance and rehabilitation assistance (5-7). Employers must also adhere to health and safety legislation, regulations and codes of practice (8,9). Those employers that manage and reduce occupational injury and disease beyond legislative demands can reduce insurance premiums, and improve productivity and company image (5,10,11). Numerous studies have identified workplace interventions as key to recovery and successful return to work, recognising that work environment factors, such as work tasks and work organisation, social relationships and organisational culture, are significant in work disability (12-16). A favourable work environment is particularly important when returning workers with mental health issues to the workplace (12).

Addressing workplace stress injury is particularly relevant in front line emergency services, such as police services. Personal and other service occupations have the highest frequency of workers' compensation claims for occupational diseases and up to 75% of these claims are for mental disorders.

Police services, corrective services and fire brigade services account for 84% of the mental disorders claims in the personal and other services occupational categories, (1), making these public order and safety occupations a primary concern for mental disorder claims. Police officers and emergency service personnel in particular face operational stressors (17,18), and these stressors are significantly added to or moderated by workplace factors (19,20), necessitating an organisational response to injury.

Organisational response to injury: Workplace rehabilitation

One response to managing the direct and indirect costs of occupational stress injury to organisations is to develop effective occupational rehabilitation systems to both prevent and manage injuries (21). Occupational rehabilitation is a process aimed at maintaining and/or restoring injured workers' functional effectiveness via appropriate and timely services (22, 23). Effective occupational rehabilitation includes immediate interventions after injury with the aim of returning injured workers back to the same workplace as early and safely as possible (5,24,25). Six essential components of successful return to work rehabilitation programs have been identified that include centralized coordination of return to work, individual psychological and occupational interventions, workplace-based interventions, work accommodations, contact between the stakeholders and concerted action (13).

While the focus of much rehabilitation literature has been on individual clinical and psychological factors associated with return to work, addressing these is not necessarily the most effective approach for promoting return to work outcomes (12-15). Whilst clinical treatment may reduce symptoms, the impact on return to work outcomes is limited unless combined with other interventions within a systems approach that acknowledges the interaction between the injured worker and health care, the work environment and the compensation system (12-14,16). Work environment factors, such as work tasks and work organisation, social relationships and organisational culture, are now recognised as significant in work disability, and numerous studies have identified workplace interventions as key to recovery and successful return to work (12-16).

Although a favourable work environment is particularly important when returning workers with mental health issues to the workplace (12), workplace interventions also have to be feasible in practice (15,16). Studies have found that implementation of return to work programs within organisations requires active participation from key stakeholders, such as injured workers and their supervisors. (15,16). Stakeholder involvement factors include interactions between all participants, including compensation, health care and the work context, recognising the multi-causality of work disability beyond the initial injury (12,13, 16). Contemporary approaches to occupational rehabilitation, such as disability management, emphasise the seamless transition from prevention to post-injury rehabilitation and the involvement of stakeholders (21,26-28).

Disability management is focused on employers and takes a systematic approach to the integration of prevention, claims management, early intervention and return to work case management (26), and has been highlighted as an effective occupational rehabilitation model, especially when applied within large organisations (21,26,28-30). Injured workers are actively involved in their rehabilitation programs and are encouraged to have input into the development of return to work goals and plans, participate in stakeholder meetings, and contribute their work experience to the design of work accommodations.

Injured workers are further empowered with information about their medical condition/s and company policies (26). This approach has been shown to achieve improvements in return to work outcomes, productivity and employee satisfaction, as well as saving on costs associated with absenteeism (26,31, 32). Large companies with successful disability management programs provide training and support for supervisors and financial incentives for departments to encourage local ownership of temporary work disability (31,32).

Supervisors, union representatives and co-workers are also actively involved in both prevention and rehabilitation processes (26). Despite the promises of a disability management approach, minimal research has been undertaken into the application of disability management policies and practices (28) and the implementation of disability management principles in organisations (30). In particular there is little published information on effective interventions in the area of occupational stress (33). Clearly there is a need for more focus on the specific needs and cultures of Australian organisations in addressing occupational rehabilitation issues.

Occupational stress

Stress and psychological injuries are of significant concern to employers due to increased workers' compensation costs, (6,30,34), and to employees given its impact on job satisfaction and quality of life (19,20,35). Physical health is also affected by chronic stress, increasing the risk of other occupational injuries to both the stressed individual and co-workers (36). Organisationally focused approaches to stress are thought to potentially benefit more employees than individually focused approaches (33), which are often now questioned in terms of their effectiveness to manage occupational stress (34,37,38). Different understandings of stress focus on different solutions, such as treating individuals or adjusting environments. Contemporary perspectives are more multidimensional than either the traditional psycho-medical or the stressor and strain model, taking ecological or systemic approaches (39). Ecologically, humans are viewed as living systems within environmental systems with psychological and social factors influencing each other (39).

In the work context, stress is best understood as a process influenced by several factors where stressors interact with an individual's capacities resulting in strain if the stressors exceed the resources (30,40). Work stress definitions are often confused by the different uses of the term stress to also denote 'stressors' (the demands), as well as 'strain' (the negative outcome of stress) (30). Perceived work stress is the extent to which a person feels strain in relation to their work. Demanding jobs that lack individual control over the work and flexibility are considered most stressful (34,41,42). However, the assumption that stress is inherently negative or that it should be completely avoided is inaccurate (43). For example positive stress that does not exceed capacity can optimise productivity, while an ongoing lack of demands to challenge an individual can lead to long term dissatisfaction and be perceived as stressful (30). Frequent work stress is most strongly associated with problems for both individuals and organisations (41). Furthermore, strain resulting from work, personal and social stressors can impact on workers and are therefore considered in work stress studies (44).

Individual versus organisational factors

Given that occupational stress is recognised as the incompatibility between individual capacity and organisational demands (30,40,44-46), it is important to address both individual and organisational causes of stress in the workplace (12,47-49). Focusing on getting a stressed worker better, only to return the worker to the same stressful workplace is clearly ineffective and therefore requires co-operation from organisational stakeholders (12). Conducting the rehabilitation process from within the workplace allows the needs of the stressed individual to be addressed in the context of simultaneous reduction in workplace stressors demonstrating the employer's commitment to the wellbeing of all workers.

Individual factors contributing to stress include those that determine ability to cope with stressors, such as personality traits and coping styles (39,50). For example, personality and locus of control have been found to affect ability to cope with interpersonal stressors (51). People with internal locus of control believe that they can influence the outcomes of a situation, whereas people with an external locus of control do not believe in their ability to control an event. Kenny (50) explores coping in the context of development from early childhood to adulthood, stating that attachment processes and other developmental experiences influence the adult personality and ability to cope with stress. Personal life stressors and life changes, such as the death of a family member, birth of a child, moving house or financial problems also generate stress that may affect ability to cope in the work context (18).

Interventions focussed on individual factors emphasise teaching individuals to control stress responses; these include behavioural self-control (52), biofeedback (53), meditation and abdominal breathing (54), progressive visualisation and cognitive processing (55). These interventions aim to decrease stress reactions by controlling thought, physiological and behavioural responses to stressors (52,53,55). Established interventions, such as cognitive behavioural therapy and psychoanalysis, have common features such as progressive visualisation and relaxation, cognitive processing, and shifting to more positive feelings and more positive behaviours (55).

Given the value of work in modern society, the amount of time spent at work and the current changes that are affecting the nature of work, it is not surprising that work stress appears to be increasing (56). Three broad 'causes' of organisational stress have been identified as job-induced (e.g., work overload), organisation-induced (e.g., communication problems) and change-induced (e.g., new supervisor) (4,57). Occupational stress and rehabilitation are impacted by organisational culture and climate, particularly in terms of how members of that organisation behave and expect others to behave (58,59). It is now clear from research that organisational climate cannot be ignored in efforts to reduce the fiscal and human costs of occupational stress (47,58).

Improving the climate (and eventually the culture) of an organisation requires supportive leadership, peer support, and a shared understanding of goals and experiences, which contributes to a positive work environment conducive to good mental health and employee motivation (47,58). Further, Bell et al. (47) suggested strategies that address organisational culture (accepting and addressing the effects of trauma), workload (adequate variety and appropriate distribution), work environment (safety and comfort), job specific education, group support (social support and debriefing opportunities), supportive supervision, and resources for self-care (counselling, support groups or other resources).

Creating healthy organisations

Given the significance of organisational factors in occupational stress, it has been proposed that the management of stress involves the creation of 'healthy organisations', which are defined as ones which recognise that health is more than the absence of stress and other ill health and therefore create an environment which facilitates good health and positive emotions (60). Healthy organisations re-focus responsibility for the health of employees to the organisation and give more control to workers by encouraging their participation in change management, job re-design, open communication, and understanding of the political or economic constraints within which the organisation operates (61). This demonstrates organisational commitment to the worker, facilitating worker commitment to the organisation. It is therefore suggested that healthy organisations are those that adopt appropriate methods of job-person matching or job design that facilitates the expertise and needs of workers; managing and rewarding performance; informing and involving workers; and supporting lifestyle and family needs of workers (60,61). According to Schurman and Israel, any organisational intervention must be specific to the context rather than 'off-the-shelf'. The intervention must engage relevant people in direct learning activities that allow them to understand stress processes in their organisation at a systemic level and should involve participants in the development of change strategies (62). Improving health and safety in a large organisation also requires good communication, a detailed analysis of needs and implementation at a systemic level with support from all areas of the organisation (57).

Police context

Over the past two decades, occupational stress literature has increasingly recognised the impact of organisational factors, such as organisational culture, on stress-related issues in policing. While police officers face operational stressors, such as occupational exposure to body fluids (17), critical incidents and violence (18), these stressors are significantly added to or moderated by organisational factors (19,20). For example, the development of PTSD, which is the most frequently investigated consequence of trauma in police officers (18), has been found to be most affected by the work environment (18,41,63).

Police stress is linked with health problems, antisocial behaviour and suicidal ideation (41,64). Causes of occupational stress for police officers include: 1) organisational factors, such as the paramilitary structures; 2) operational issues associated with tasks such as protecting people, rescuing traumatised people, role conflicts and dangerous work; 3) external systems, such as the criminal justice system, and public perceptions, including media coverage and; 4) personal life stressors (18). Critical incidents are defined as adverse events, which may result in a range of symptoms from exhaustion to symptoms of progressing mental illness (63). These have been linked with post-traumatic stress disorder (PTSD) symptoms in police officers, including measurable physical and physiological symptoms (18,20,63). Indeed, police officers are exposed to a high degree of work stress in the form of critical incidents and 'disasters', such as intentional violence against humans, and studies have therefore linked police work to conditions such as "vicarious traumatization, secondary traumatic stress, traumatic counter transference, burnout, and compassion fatigue" (18).

The situation of workplace stress for police is more complex than the stress relating to critical incidents, thereby requiring attention to a range of psychological, organisational and operational factors. Police work stressors are often described as organisational (such as lack of recognition) and operational (such as dealing with the public) (18,63). Psychological characteristics such as an external locus of control and negative affect have been linked to increased occupational stress experiences in correctional officers (65). Similarly, ineffective coping mechanisms, such as avoidance, are strongly related to perceived work stress and health outcomes, such as anxiety and burnout in police officers (41). In addition to the individual factors linked with poor mental health outcomes, police officers have complex work environments, including inadequate equipment, unsuitable co-workers, unfair workload distribution, inadequate supervision, unclear work roles, and shift work (41,63).

According to Mayhew (19), health and safety risks in policing include critical incidents, such as death, homicide and assault on police officers. However, this list of risks also includes organisational factors such as stress and fatigue due to staff shortages, limited job control, staff conflict, autocratic management, unfair performance appraisal, workers' compensation tribunal hearings and police culture (19), as well as poor relationships and lack of internal communication (20,66). Numerous studies indicate that work environment stress, rather than critical incidents, best predict perceived stress, PTSD symptoms and other health problems (41,63). Work environment stressors include a lack of consultation and communication, inadequate control and excessive workloads, and poor levels of support (63). Organisational stressors and the negative public image of the police have also been found to magnify the impact of critical incidents faced by police officers (67). Outside of the workplace, negative life events, including work-family conflict, and past trauma also contribute to PTSD symptoms (63).

Mental health problems, including PTSD symptoms, in police officers have been linked to four factors: 1) regular exposure to traumatic events; 2) an individual's previous exposure to trauma; 3) "negative life events" outside of work; and 4) "routine work environment stress" (63). Maguen et al. acknowledge that policing is stressful and results in both physical and psychological symptoms. They examined the links between 'routine work environment stress' and PTSD symptoms utilising several measures of the four factors listed above to assess 180 recruits and reassess them after 12 months on the job. They found that the fourth factor (routine work environment stress) was most closely linked to PTSD symptoms. Work environment stressors affecting PTSD symptoms included dysfunctional equipment, routine operational hassles, work role ambiguity, poor interpersonal relationships with co-workers and discrimination (63).

There is a strong association between policing work and traumatic stress and burnout (18,20,63). There are also behavioural impacts of chronic stress among police officers, including suicide, drug and alcohol abuse, absenteeism and premature retirement, all of which occur at significantly higher rates than in other occupational groups (19,68). These findings have prompted research and discussion focused on addressing these risks in the police context. For instance, social support has been found to protect against the development of burnout and traumatisation conditions in police (18), and this extends to social support from the workplace. A supportive work environment protects police officers from developing PTSD symptoms and other mental health problems, by providing a compassionate context within which critical incidents are processed. Workplace cohesion and morale and strong leadership improve role clarity and job engagement and protects against the effects of stress (63). Furthermore, the workplace mediates between negative life events outside of work and PTSD symptoms. It was therefore concluded that whilst the organisation cannot control critical incidents and negative life events, it can provide the environment to buffer against the impacts of these factors (63). Prior trauma was also dismissed as a significant predictor of PTSD, suggesting that the focus should be on optimising the work environment rather than assessing previous traumatic events in police recruits' lives (63).

Occupational rehabilitation challenges in police organisations

Police organisations need to address the complex issue of occupational stress due to the psychological, physical and behavioural impact of this occupational illness on individuals and their organisation. However, despite the significant body of evidence implicating organisational factors in the cause of occupational stress in policing, prevention activities (such as initial and ongoing police training) have continued to focus on operational dangers, leaving police officers ill prepared for organisational stressors (20,66). This imbalance between the evidence about causes of mental health conditions in police work and the interventions focused on treating individuals, rather than changing the organisational environment, has been echoed by other stress research (18,41). Accordingly, Gershon et al. (41) recommend a multi-layered approach, aimed at improving coping mechanisms in officers (shifting from avoidant and negative coping strategies to cognitive problem-solving strategies), as well as addressing modifiable stressors such as organisational unfairness and job dissatisfaction. They also describe innovative strategies implemented by some progressive police organisations that include provision of specific cognitive problem solving skills programs, Alcoholics Anonymous groups, couples' counselling retreats, peer support programs, changes to organisational structure, improved training programs and critical incident management systems (41).

Prevention and rehabilitation processes are likely to be affected by the police personality and culture. Police working personalities are developed in the context of the paramilitary organisational culture, the divided organisational subcultures (officers and staff) and the nature of their duties (69,70). These working personalities have been found to include characteristics such as natural suspicion (of outsiders and management), increased alertness to danger, solidarity with other serving officers and bravery (71-73). In the policing context, injury or disease translates to no longer being an active serving officer, no longer being seen as brave and not being able to stand alongside colleagues in the face of danger; these 'signs of weakness' stand in direct contrast to the accepted behaviour of police officers. In summary, the contextual and process issues described above suggest that solutions need to be sought in both overt processes and policies, and less tangible interpersonal factors concerning organisational culture, climate, characteristics and understandings about stress.

Addressing occupational stress in police organisations

Consistent with an ecological focus on addressing occupational stress in police the following recommendations reflect the complex nature of this condition. Changes to the organisational culture of police services, from the prevailing 'macho'/ paramilitary environment, would positively impact on injury prevention and early intervention efforts, encouraging members to remain positively engaged with their organisations. Research from the past 20 years indicates that organisational climate cannot be ignored in efforts to reduce the fiscal and human costs of occupational stress (47,58). Addressing the punitive culture of police organisations is necessary to prevent general bullying, particularly of injured and recovering workers. Organisational culture is often a cause of police officers' hesitation in reporting stress related issues, which limits the organisation's capacity to respond to problems and implement effective and early secondary prevention and rehabilitation. Improving the climate (and eventually the culture) of an organisation requires supportive leadership, peer support, and a shared understanding of goals and experiences, which contributes to a positive work environment conducive to good mental health and employee motivation (47,58). Trust is an important issue in organisational culture, and is built upon a shared identity between supervisors and supervisees and ongoing co-operation between them (74).

Consistent with a disability management approach to managing injury, staff at all levels of the organisation should be involved in strategy development and supporting health, wellbeing and rehabilitation initiatives. Lack of worker involvement in these areas reduces the potential for prevention and rehabilitation (75), with failures to develop healthy organisations attributed to the fact that change was not managed with the participation of the workers (62). Healthy organisations re-focus the responsibility for health to the organisation, but simultaneously give more control to workers by encouraging their participation in change management, job re-design, open communication, and understanding of the political or economic constraints within which the organisation operates (60,61).

Dissemination of information to promote understanding about prevention and rehabilitation within the police service is critical to successful rehabilitation initiatives. This includes: (a) information about the prevention and rehabilitation of physical and psychological injury and illness for specific members of the organisation; (b) supervisors to be more informed about stress issues, prevention and rehabilitation to undertake their role in making decisions and providing support for staff; (c) clearer boundaries between industrial relations issues and rehabilitation; (d) better understanding by injured workers of rehabilitation procedures, and the roles of support staff; and (e) more information and support for the families of injured and stressed officers.

Organisations must adopt a more holistic and comprehensive understanding of psychological issues, including personal stressors. This is consistent with research that showed whilst both individual and organisational factors influenced the development of vicarious trauma, the focus of intervention remained on affected individuals (47). Practically useful website information designed for officers, including flow charts, contact details and useful links, should be provided and regularly promoted to all stakeholders so they are more informed and confident in the rehabilitation process. Supervisors need training to detect early signs of stress to prevent the escalation of mental health issues to dangerous levels, as well as understanding and supporting different coping mechanisms. People in support roles need knowledge and skills to effectively manage rehabilitation, including advanced people management and communication skills. It is important that there are clear requirements and processes for all stakeholders when injured workers returned to the workplace. Advice to injured workers about what to expect during the return to work process and education for others in that workplace allows for more realistic expectations and more positive return to work experiences. Resources for self-care, such as counselling, support groups or other resources, have also been identified as important to maintaining wellbeing within an organisation (47).

A critical component of occupational rehabilitation for police officers is the availability of systematic debriefing processes that are automatically initiated and adequately resourced to prevent subsequent psychological issues. Research suggests that a supportive work environment protects police officers from developing PTSD symptoms and other mental health problems, by providing a compassionate context within which critical incidents are processed. Workplace cohesion and morale and strong leadership improve role clarity and job engagement and protects against the effects of stress (63). Furthermore, the workplace mediates between negative life events outside of work and PTSD symptoms.

Interventions are required at each stage of the occupational rehabilitation process from pre-injury through to maintenance of the return to work. There are several potential improvements to be made to develop more proactive and strategic injury and illness prevention initiatives. A feature of a comprehensive disability management approach to occupational stress is the ongoing data collection and evaluation of the common causes of stress, injury and attrition to improve prevention systems and strategies for serving officers. Upon identifying a problematic area for injuries and illness, the issues should be followed up and addressed in consultation with local managers. Simpson (4) recommends systematic organisational assessment of risks considering all levels, including the whole organisation, work groups and individuals, to effectively address organisational needs.

As a pre-injury strategy organisations should develop a detailed understanding of job factors and organisational characteristics that can be used to counteract the sometimes unavoidable operational risk factors associated with policing, particularly those causing mental illness, such as PTSD. Reducing work environment stressors and improving organisational support mechanisms reduces the development of serious mental illness, despite the operational risks. Further, improving training and knowledge for key stakeholders and providers may stem the escalation of stress, reduce the impact of injury and improve the outcomes of rehabilitation. A better awareness of stress and injury management processes for all stakeholders can improve the social structures and actions of officers to increase trust in the organisation and understanding about prevention and rehabilitation, thereby reducing the negative influence of stigma. Increased awareness requires time, resources and genuine interest in training to create a context where individuals feel more comfortable in reporting stress and participating in rehabilitation processes. Providing occupational rehabilitation awareness training can therefore have a broad and far reaching impact on injury prevention and rehabilitation outcomes in the organisation.

Injury and illness reporting processes are affected by the organisational climate, trust issues, as well as understanding of stress and rehabilitation processes. The needs and experiences of injured and ill individuals therefore need to take precedence over formal procedures to increase officers' willingness to seek help for stress or other issues impacting work capacity. Training to recognise stress and strategies to compensate for geographic isolation are required to identify absences and initiate earlier rehabilitation. Once a rehabilitation need is identified, stakeholders need simple clear processes to fast track reporting and initiate support, especially when there is no workers' compensation claim to guide the process. To achieve an increase in the rate of reporting of stress and other illness, strategies have to be approached in a supportive manner and be combined with making leaders more accountable for their people management skills and preparing the leaders of the future for this aspect of the role. Non-judgemental support and information about processes, such as lodging a workers' compensation claim, encourages people to report stress symptoms and obtain early assistance.

Effective systems for early identification of stress and wellbeing issues can prevent injuries. Absenteeism management strategies include identifying non-consecutive absence patterns that might point to early signs of stress, training for supervisors to identify and respond to issues before they escalate, and improved secondary prevention systems, including risk management and debriefing after traumatic incidents. These changes require a shift in the prevailing social structures that expect police officers to get on with the job regardless of what they have experienced. If the damage is psychological, individuals should receive appropriate care and treatment, such as mental health first aid. People in support and supervisory roles need work structures that allow them to get to know staff to be able to detect potential stress and rehabilitation issues, and respond before early signs of stress escalate to serious psychological injury.

An effective approach for responding to injury is the removal of the distinction between compensable and non-compensable cases, streamlining processes and clarifying responsibilities for responding to injury, and focusing on achieving optimal outcomes and addressing individual needs. Both external and internal factors influence organisations, creating tension between people and processes. Whilst compensable cases tend to have some clear processes driven by the workers' compensation authority, they create complexities in other organisational processes, such as the transition from the workers' compensation decision to internal support mechanisms. At the initial contact with the absent individual, an increased focus on addressing needs will reduce the risk of a non-compensable case being dismissed as needing no support at all. Similarly, when a workers' compensation claim is rejected by the insurer internal support options should still be considered, because a workers' compensation claim may be rejected based on eligibility criteria even if the individual needs support for an illness that affects their ability to work. For example, a drop in the number of mental stress claims has been linked to jurisdictions tightening up on what is accepted, thereby reducing claim numbers but not the incidence of stress (76,77). More proactive intervention outside of the claims process and would increase officers' trust in the organisation that they will be looked after following injury.

Streamlining processes and clarifying responsibilities for responding to injury, illness and absence is important to facilitate intervention and is required to increase trust in the organisation, increase local ownership of rehabilitation, and improve rehabilitation outcomes. This should include simplifying processes for interaction with external stakeholders like the workers' compensation authority and streamlining processes to initiate early intervention. Responding processes need to be focused on achieving optimal outcomes and addressing individual needs. The initial direct contact with the affected member needs to be early to gain an overview of the affected officer's needs and achieve a successful return to work. This requires minimal barriers to reporting. Injured workers need to be directly involved in communication throughout the rehabilitation process. Promoting individual ownership of rehabilitation has been established as important (26), and includes mechanisms encouraging feedback about support processes. Good communication with the absent officer early in the process helps them to understand issues, processes, roles and responsibilities, and promotes their constructive participation in the rehabilitation process. Early and effective contact with the absent individual is an opportunity to re-establish or maintain the occupational bond, address tensions and reduce stressors (30). If the initial contact is delayed or ineffective due to lack of time or excessive focus on paperwork, the whole rehabilitation process is jeopardised.

Intervention processes need to be focused on well-established principles of effective rehabilitation, especially for people with mental health problems. For instance, a holistic bio-psychosocial approach with multidisciplinary input, cognitive behavioural therapy and organisational interventions has been found to be effective in improving mental health and promoting successful return to work (78). Provided specific organisational needs are addressed, appropriate individual interventions are provided and stakeholder participation strategies are effectively implemented, well integrated return to work programs have been found to be effective for a range of conditions (12-16). Investing in rehabilitation interventions is cost effective because it promotes return to work outcomes and reduces compensation costs. Interventions aimed at return to work focus on job accommodations, including modified work tasks and work organisation (12,13). Creative approaches to finding return to work options for people requiring suitable duties are enhanced by easily accessible job descriptions and involving injured employees in decision-making. Van Oostrom et al. (15) found that facilitating injured workers and supervisors to develop their own consensus-based solutions to return to work barriers is effective in identifying obstacles and practical solutions. The roles of supervisors and co-workers in a successful return to work process are vital, especially when mental health problems are involved, but these stakeholders often lack the knowledge and skills required to fulfil this role effectively, jeopardising the return to work outcome (12). As the return to work process is quite dependent on support from supervisors, they need to be well informed. Other stakeholders in the workplace, such as co-workers, also need information about the return to work process to be able to accommodate the limitations prescribed on suitable duties plans. A favourable work environment is particularly important when returning workers with mental health issues to the workplace (12).

Return to work maintenance needs attention to achieve complete resolution of issues. In some cases the organisation should be more flexible about rehabilitation goals if permanently modified duties make the return to work more sustainable. For psychological and serious injuries there is a particular need for procedural mechanisms to ensure return to work maintenance and resolution of issues. Such mechanisms include systems to detect a re-emergence of health issues early and to restart the rehabilitation process quickly to ensure continued work functioning. Long-term monitoring, especially for psychological illnesses, is beneficial. In particular, all stakeholders within the workplace need to have an understanding of the long-term nature of mental health issues to support long-term return to work maintenance.

Conclusion

It is evident in Australia that there are ongoing challenges for the management of workplace stress stemming from workers' compensation and organisational systems. Rising costs associated with workplace injury and illness, especially as a result of mental stress, indicate the need for research that focuses on the specific occupational rehabilitation needs and practices of large organisations, taking into account the complex interactions between individual and organisational factors. In policing organisations, there is a particular need to consider the organisational climate and culture and to address these with input from all levels of the organisation. While effective processes and policies are important, interpersonal factors concerning organisational culture, climate, characteristics and understandings about stress need to be understood and managed. Effective organisational communication is required to address both interpersonal and organisational issues and achieve a balance between the two. Creating a healthy organisational environment capable of identifying and addressing the needs of officers, improving the organisational climate to increase reporting of health concerns, and responding to and addressing injury or illness with a focus on individual needs will contribute to achieving more sustainable return to work outcomes. Effective occupational rehabilitation systems in police services therefore require insight into interpersonal factors and organisational processes to address established social structures and the actions of officers, as well as the interactions between them.

References

[1] Safe Work Australia. Compendium of workers' compensation statistics Australia 2009-10. In: Section DA, editor. Canberra: Safe Work Australia, 2012:111.

[2] Jauregui M, Schnall PL. Work, psychosocial stressors, and the bottom line. In: Schnall PL, Dobson M, Rosskam E, eds. Unhealthy work: causes, consequences, cures. Critical approaches in the health social sciences series. Amityville, NY: Baywood, 2009:153-67.

[3] Working Carers Gateway. Managing stress in the workplace Lismore: NSW Health, 2010. Accessed 2013 Mar 10. URL: http://www.workingcarers.org.au/work/1149-managing-stress-at-work-for-employers-and-employees.

[4] Simpson B. Occupational stress: Assessing the risk, addressing the hazard. In: Barrett T, Cameron D, eds. Safe business, good business A practical guide to occupational safety, health and insurance in Australasia, 2 ed. Guildford, Western Australia: Vinyard Publishing, 2004:151-69.

[5] WorkCover Queensland. Insurance Brisbane: WorkCover Queensland, 2012. Accessed 2013 Mar 10. URL: http://www.workcoverqld.com.au/insurance.
[6] Biggs HC. Occupational concerns and workplace well-health. Work 2009;32(1):1-3.
[7] Department of Industrial Relations Queensland. What are your obligations? General information, 2005.
[8] Department of Justice and Attorney-General. What are your obligations? General information. [Government website]. The State of Queensland, 2010. Accessed 2013 Mar 10. URL: http://www.deir.qld.gov.au/workplace/rights/yourobligation/info/index.htm.
[9] National Research Centre for Occupational Health and Safety Regulation. About occupational health and safety regulation in Australia [University website]. Canberra: Australian National University, 2002. funded by WorkCover NSW, WorkSafe Victoria and Workplace Health and Safety Queensland]. Accessed 2013 Mar 10. URL: http://ohs.anu.edu.au/ohs/index.php.
[10] CCH Occupational Health and Safety. Workplace rehabilitation manual Safety COH, editor. North Ryde, NSW: CCH Australia, 1990.
[11] NOHSC. The cost of work-related injury and illness for Australian employers, workers and the community. Canberra: NOHSC, Commonwealth of Australia, 2004.
[12] Briand C, Durand M-J, St-Arnaud L, Corbière M. Work and mental health: Learning from return-to-work rehabilitation programs designed for workers with musculoskeletal disorders. Int J Law Psychiatry 2007;30(4-5):444-57.
[13] Briand C, Durand M-J, St-Arnaud L, Corbière M. How well do return-to-work interventions for musculoskeletal conditions address the multicausality of work disability? J Occup Rehabil 2008;18(2):207-17.
[14] Wald J, Taylor S. Work impairment and disability in Posttraumatic Stress Disorder: A review and recommendations for psychological injury research and practice. Psychol Inj Law 2009;2(3):254-62.
[15] van Oostrom S, van Mechelen W, Terluin B, de Vet H, Anema J. A participatory workplace intervention for employees with distress and lost time: A feasibility evaluation within a Randomized Controlled Trial. J Occup Rehabil 2009;19(2):212-22.
[16] Tjulin Å, Edvardsson Stiwne E, Ekberg K. Experience of the implementation of a multi-stakeholder return-to-work programme. J Occup Rehabil 2009;19(4):409-18.
[17] Wald J. The psychological consequences of occupational blood and body fluid exposure injuries. Disabil Rehabil 2009;31(23):1963-9.
[18] Patterson GT. Mental stress and workers' compensation claims among police officers. J Workplace Rights 2009;14(4):441-55.
[19] Mayhew C. Occupational health and safety risks faced by police officers. Canberra: Australian Institute of Criminology, 2001.
[20] Stinchcomb J. Searching for stress in all the wrong places: Combating chronic organisational stressors in policing. Pol Prac Res 2004;5(3):259-77.
[21] Harder H, Scott L. Comprehensive disability management. Edinburgh: Elsevier, 2005.
[22] WorkCover NSW. Glossary. 2003.

[23] NOHSC. Uniform guidelines for accreditation of rehabilitation providers. Canberra: Australian Government Publishing Service, 1995.
[24] Harrison K, Allen S. Features of occupational rehabilitation systems in Australia: A map through the maze. Work 2003;21(2):141-52.
[25] WorkCover NSW. Workers compensation and injury management fact sheet 2: Injury management and return-to-work programs. In: WorkCoverNSW, ed. Gosford, NSW: WorkCover NSW; no date.
[26] Buys N, Randall C. Disability management: A global response to disability in the workplace. In: Marshall C, Kendall E, Banks M, Gover RM, eds. Disabilities: Insights from across fields and around the world. Westport, CT: Praeger, 2009: 129-44.
[27] Smith D. Implementing disability management: A review of basic concepts and essential components. Empl Assist Quart 1997;12(4):37-50.
[28] Westmorland M, Buys N. Disability management in a sample of Australian self-insured companies. Disabil Rehabil 2002;24(14):746-54.
[29] Shrey D. Disability management in industry: the new paradigm in injured worker rehabilitation. Disabil Rehabil 1996;18(8):408-14.
[30] Kendall E, Muenchberger H. Stress at work: Using a process model to assist employers to understand the trajectory. Work 2009;32(1):19-25.
[31] Ceniceros R. Disability accommodation programs cut costs. Business Insurance 2010;44(33):24.
[32] McDonald C. Integrated disability management fuels power company's comp claim success. National Underwriter PC 2010;114(29):12-3, 27.
[33] Caulfield N, Chang D, Dollard MF, Elshaug C. A review of occupational stress interventions in Australia. Int J Stress Manage 2004;11(2):149-66.
[34] Kompier M, Taris T. Psychosocial risk factors and work-related issues: state of the art and issues for future research. In: Antoniou A-S, Cooper C, eds. Research companion to organizational health psychology. New horizons in management. Cheltenham, UK: Edward Elgar Publishing, 2005:59-69.
[35] Graves W. Police cynicism: Causes and cures. FBI Law Enforc Bull 1996;65:16-20.
[36] Dollard M. Introduction: Context, theories and intervention In: Dollard M, Winefield A, Winefield H, eds. Occupational stress in the service professions London: Taylor Francis, 2003:1-42.
[37] Dick P. The social construction of the meaning of acute stressors: A qualitative study of the personal accounts of police officers using a stress counselling service. Work Stress 2000;14(3):226-44.
[38] Hart PM, Cotton P. Conventional wisdom is often misleading: police stress within an organisational health framework. In: Dollard MF, Winefield AH, Winefield HR, eds. Occupational stress in the service professions. London: Taylor Francis, 2003: 103–41.
[39] Kenny D, McIntyre D. Constructions of occupational stress: nuisances, nuances or novelties. In: Antoniou A-S, Cooper C, eds. Research companion to organizational health psychology. New horizons in management. Cheltenham, UK: Edward Elgar Publishing, 2005:20-58.

[40] Gordon DR, Schnall PL. Beyond the individual: Connecting work environment and health. In: Schnall PL, Dobson M, Rosskam E, eds. Unhealthy work: Causes, consequences, cures. Critical approaches in the health social sciences. New York: Baywood, 2009:1-15.

[41] Gershon RRM, Barocas B, Canton AN, Li X, Vlahov D. Mental, physical, and behavioral outcomes associated with perceived work stress in police officers. Crim Justice Behav 2009;36(3):275-89.

[42] Spooner-Lane R, Patton W. Determinants of burnout among public hospital nurses. Aust J Adv Nurs 2007;25(1):8-16.

[43] Nelson D, Simmons B. Eustress and attitudes at work: a positive approach. In: Antoniou A-S, Cooper C, editors. Research companion to organizational health psychology. New horizons in management. Cheltenham, UK: Edward Elgar Publishing, 2005:102-10.

[44] Kendall E, Muenchberger H. Stressors and supports across work and non-work domains: The impact on mental health and the workplace. Work 2009;32(1):27-37.

[45] Diamantopoulou A. Europe under stress. Work Stress 2002;5:3.

[46] Humphrey J. Job Stress. Needman Heights, MA: Allyn Bacon, 1998.

[47] Bell H, Kulkarni S, Dalton L. Organizational prevention of vicarious trauma. Fam Society 2003;84(4):463-70.

[48] Giga SI, Cooper CL, Faragher B. The development of a framework for a comprehensive approach to stress management interventions at work. Int J Stress Manage 2003;10(4):280-96.

[49] La Montagne AD. Evaluation of occupational stress interventions: An overview. National Occupational Health and Safety Commission Symposium on the OH&S implications of stress, 12 December 2001; Melbourne: National Occupational Health Safety Commission, 2001.

[50] Kenny D. Psychological foundations of stress and coping: A developmental perspective. In: Kenny DT, Carlson JG, McGuigan FJ, Sheppard JL, eds. Stress and health: Research and clinical applications. Australia: Harwood Academic, 2000:73-104.

[51] Hahn SE. The effects of locus of control on daily exposure, coping and reactivity to work interpersonal stressors: a diary study. Pers Individ Dif 2000;29(4):729-48.

[52] McGuigan FJ. Why might stress management methods be effective? In: Kenny DT, Carlson JG, McGuigan FJ, Sheppard JL, eds. Stress and health: research and clinical applications. Australia: Harwood Academic, 2000:151-61.

[53] McKee MG, Kiffer JF. Biofeedback and stress. In: Kenny DT, Carlson JG, McGuigan FJ, Sheppard JL, eds. Stress and health: research and clinical applications. Australia: Harwood Academic, 2000:163-78.

[54] Stoyva J. Stress management: What can we learn from the meditative disciplines? In: Kenny DT, Carlson JG, McGuigan FJ, Sheppard JL, eds. Stress and health: research and clinical applications. Australia: Harwood Academic, 2000:179-93.

[55] Sheppard JL. Behavior change following affect shift: A model for the treatment of stress disorders. In: Kenny DT, Carlson JG, McGuigan FJ, Sheppard JL, eds. Stress and health: research and clinical applications. Australia: Harwood Academic, 2000:195-222.

[56] Szymanski EM. Disability, job stress, the changing nature of careers, and the career resilience portfolio. Rehabil Couns Bull 1999;42:279-84.

[57] Kendall E, Murphy P, Bursnall S, O'Neill V. Containing the costs of occupational stress: A new approach to identifying, defining, preventing and managing stress in the workplace. Perth: Workcover WA, 2001.

[58] Cotton P. Developing an optimal organisational climate. Towards safest workplaces II, March 2004: ComCare; 2004.

[59] Muchinsky P. Psychology applied to work: An introduction to industrial and organisational psychology, 5th ed. Pacific Grove CA: Brookes/Cole, 1997.

[60] Cartwright S, Cooper C. The role of organizations in promoting health and wellbeing. In: Cartwright S, Cooper C, eds. Innovations in stress and health. Basingstoke: Palgrave Macmillan, 2011:153-72.

[61] Henry J. The healthy organization. In: Antoniou A-S, Cooper C, eds. Research companion to organizational health psychology. New horizons in management. Cheltenham, UK: Edward Elgar Publishing, 2005:382-92.

[62] Schurman S, Israel B. Redesigning work systems to reduce stress: A participatory action research approach to creating change. In: Murphy L, Hurrell J, Sauter S, Keita G, eds. Job Stress Interventions. Washington, DC: American Psychological Association, 1995.

[63] Maguen S, Metzler TJ, McCaslin SE, Inslicht SS, Henn-Haase C, Neylan TC, et al. Routine work environment stress and PTSD symptoms in police officers. J Nerv Ment Dis 2009;197(10):754-60.

[64] Collins PA, Gibbs ACC. Stress in police officers: a study of the origins, prevalence and severity of stress-related symptoms within a county police force. Occup Med 2003;53(4):256-64.

[65] Botha C, Pienaar J. South African correctional official occupational stress: the role of psychological strengths. J Crim Justice 2006;34(1):73-84.

[66] Kop N, Euwema M, Schaufeli W. Burnout, job stress and violent behaviour among Dutch police officers. Work Stress 1999;13(4):326-40.

[67] Brown J, Fielding J, Grover J. Distinguishing traumatic, vicarious and routine operational stressor exposure and attendant adverse consequences in a sample of police officers. Work Stress 1999;13(4):312-25.

[68] Anshel MH, Robertson M, Caputi P. Sources of acute stress and their appraisals and reappraisals among Australian police as a function of previous experience. J Occup Org Psych 1997;70(4):337-56.

[69] Parsons D, Jesilow P. In the same voice: Women and men in law enforcement. Santa Ana, CA: Seven Locks Press, 2001.

[70] Perez DW, Shtull PR. Police research and practice: An American perspective. Police Pract Res 2002;3(3):169-87.

[71] Skolnick J. A sketch of the police officer's "working personality". In: Hancock B, Sharp PM, eds. Criminal justice in America: Theory, practice and policy. Upper Saddle River, NJ: Prentice Hall, 1996.

[72] Kappeler VE, Sluder RD, Alpert GP. Forces of deviance: Understanding the dark side of policing. Prospect Heights, IL: Waveland Press, 1994.

[73] Prenzler T. Is there a police culture? Aust J Public Admin 1997;54(4):47-56.

[74] Dirks K, Skarlicki D. Trust in leaders: Existing research and emerging issues. In: Kramer R, Cook K, eds. Trust and distrust in organizations: Dilemmas and approaches. New York: Russell Sage Foundation, 2004:21-40.
[75] O'Donnell C. Motor accident and workers' compensation insurance design for high quality health outcomes and cost containment. Disabil Rehabil 2000;22:88-96.
[76] Safe Work Australia. Compendium of workers' compensation statistics Australia 2008–09. In: Section DA, ed. Canberra: Safe Work Australia, 2011.
[77] Safe Work Australia. Work-related injuries in Australia, 2005–06: Factors affecting applications for workers' compensation Canberra: Commonwealth of Australia, 2009.
[78] Campbell J, Wright C, Moseley A, Chilvers R, Richards S, Stabb L. Avoiding long-term incapacity for work: Developing an early intervention in primary care. Exeter, UK: Peninsula Medical School, Primary Care Research Group, 2007.

SECTION TWO: QUALITY OF LIFE, STUDENTS AND GREEN TEA

In: Health Promotion
Editors: J. Sun, N. Buys, J. Merrick
ISBN: 978-1-62257-870-2

Chapter IV

Using the Illinois Test of Psycholinguistic Ability to assess visual and auditory abilities in Chinese children with learning difficulties

Jing Sun, PhD [*1] ***and Nicholas Buys, PhD*** [2]
[1]School of Public Health and Griffith Health Institute, Griffith University, Gold Coast Campus, Parkland, Australia
[2]School of Human Services and Social Work, and Griffith Health Institute, Griffith University, Parkland, Gold Coast, Australia

Abstract

There is ample evidence to indicate that children with learning difficulties have visual-perceptual and auditory ability deficits. The aim of this chapter was to investigate whether the deficits in visual-perceptual and auditory abilities also exist in Chinese children in the schools. One-

[*] *Correspondence:* Jing Sun, PhD, School of Public Health, Griffith University and Griffith Health Institute, Griffith University, Gold Coast Campus, Parkland, Q4222 Australia. E-mail: j.sun@griffith.edu.au

hundred-forty nine students aged 6 to 10 years who attended Child Growth and Development Clinics at Capital Institute of Pediatrics, Beijing, China were invited to attend the study, and 54 children who had no learning difficulties and had normal neurological development were randomly selected from the local schools as the control group. The results showed significant lower scores in visual-perceptual and auditory abilities in the study group than control group. To prevent children's learning difficulties, health promotion focusing on visual-perceptual and auditory abilities should be mandatory for children who have learning difficulties, even in the absence of neurological impairments and with normal general intelligence development.

Introduction

Although children with learning disabilities are often regarded as a heterogeneous group, they often have difficulties in processing information using their visual-perceptual and auditory abilities. Their visual and auditory abilities are related to the academic performance of students with learning disabilities (1). Research on the relationship of visual and auditory abilities to learning disabilities is often associated with the constructs of comprehension, memory, association, and integration of visual and auditory abilities, and visual and verbal expression (1-3). Mammarella (3) and colleagues found children with learning difficulties had spatial working memory deficits compared to normal matched counterparts. A recent study by Menghini and colleagues (4) found children with dyslexia had difficulties not only in comprehension and phonological coding, but also visual spatial working memory.

Other studies found the occurrence of learning difficulties in children in reading, maths and written language was related to the deficits of spatial-visual abilities (5). Despite ample findings of visual and auditory deficits in children with learning difficulties, there are no studies that have assessed these deficits in Chinese children with learning difficulties. This study explores the characteristics of visual and auditory abilities among Chinese children with learning disabilities.

Our study

One hundred and forty five children with learning difficulties, 103 male (69.1%) and 42 female (31.9%), were recruited from Child Growth and Development Clinics at the Affiliated Children's Hospital in Capital Institute of Pediatrics in Beijing, China. The subjects were referred for evaluation by teachers because of their low academic performance, behavioral and/or learning problems. Subjects with known neurological disorders including epilepsy, traumatic brain injury, and neurological impairments were excluded from the study. The criteria for the inclusion of children as subjects in the study group were: 1) the children's school achievement was below the 10% percentile based on grade level, 2) the children's level or intelligence was within the normal range or above average and 3) there were no visual and hearing impairments (examined by the neurologists at Children's Hospital of Capital Institute of Pediatrics, Beijing, China). All children were from families of Han ethnic origin and from middle to low socio-economic levels. Fifty two children aged 6 to 10 years who had normal academic achievement and normal intelligence scores on the Wechsler Intelligence Test were randomly chosen from children from grades one to four from a local primary school as the comparison group. The informed consents were obtained from parents of the participating children. The ethical clearance to conduct the study was approved by the research board of the Capital Institute of Pediatrics, Beijing, China.

Measures

The ITPA subtests were used to assess visual and auditory abilities of the children (6, 7). These subtests are designed to assess fundamental abilities underlying learning process by sampling three dimensions, i.e., two channels of communication (auditory-vocal, visual-motor), psycholinguistic processes (reception, association, expression), and levels of organization (representational, automatic). The ITPA consists of 10 subtests, including Auditory Reception, Visual Reception, Auditory Association, Visual Association , Verbal Expression , Manual Expression, Grammatic Closure, Visual Closure, Auditory Sequential Memory, and Visual Sequential Memory. The reliability and validity of ITPA test is high with internal consistency coefficients range from .60-.96, with a median of .88 (7). Information regarding demographic data including age, gender, type of family, living condition was collected using a questionnaire. Information relating to parental education methods, parity, child's sleeping status, type of delivery, size of accommodation, birth weight, and time length of lack of oxygen was also collected.

Statistical methods

Comparisons of differences between study and control groups on demographic variables, family functioning, disease history, birth status, were conducted using Chi-square for the categorical variables, and t test for continuous variables. An independent sample t test was used to compare the difference between study and control groups in visual-perceptual and auditory abilities. To explore the correlation between visual and auditory abilities, a Pearson correlation test was used. For all statistical tests, statistical significance was accepted as at probability (P value) level less than 0.05.

Our findings

Table 1 demonstrates that there are significant differences between study and control groups in gender, parental education methods, and living conditions.

Table 1. Comparison of demographic factors between study and control group

Variables	Normal child (N= 54)	Child with learning disability (N= 149)	Chi-square value	P
	N (%)	N (%)		
Gender				
Female	24 (48.0%)	44 (29.9%)	5.39	0.02
Male	26 (52.0%)	103 (70.1)		
Type of family				
Single parent	1 (2.0%)	3 (2.1%)	4.80	0.30
Nuclear family	23 (46.0%)	82 (56.6%)		
Big family with grandparents	18 (36.0%)	37 (25.5%)		

Variables	Normal child (N= 54)	Child with learning disability (N= 149)	Chi-square value	P
Big family which had more than two Nuclear family	5 (10.0)	7 (4.8%)		
Grandparent living with grandchildren	3 (6.0%)	16 (11.0%)		
Method of education of parents				
Over protective, spoiling, lenient and superseding	3 (6.1%)	22 (15.1%)	15.92	0.001
Simple, rigid and autocratic	5 (10.2%)	30 (20.5%)		
Democratic, patient and teach with skill and patience	22 (44.9%)	26 (17.8%)		
Inconsistent methods	19 (38.8%)	68 (46.6%)		
Accommodation Type				
House	26 (54.2%)	44 (30.8%)	8.47	0.004
Apartment	22 (45.8 %)	99 (69.2%)		
Child sleep with parent				
Independent sleeping	9 (18.8%)	35 (24.0%)	2.94	0.23
sleep with somebody	22 (45.8%)	47 (32.2%)		
sleep with parents	17 (35.4%)	64 (43.8%)		
Prenatal Diseases				
Yes	4 (8.5%)	11 (8.0%)	0.01	0.92
No	43 (91.5%)	126 (92.0%)		
Prenatal diseases				
1	5 (38.5%)	20 (40.8%)	7.28	0.20
2	0 (0.0%)	2 (4.1%)		
3	3 (23.1%)	16 (32.7%)		
4	3 (23.1%)	5 (10.2%)		
8	2 (15.3%)	1 (2.0%)		
10	0 (0.0%)	5 (10.2%)		
Gravida				
1	36 (78.3%)	90 (72.0%)	0.96	0.81
2	8 (17.4%)	28 (22.4%)		
3	2 (4.3%)	6 (4.8%)		
4	0 (0.0%)	1 (0.8%)		
Parity				
1	43 (100.0%)	116 (96.7%)	1.47	0.48
2	0 (0.0%)	3 (2.5%)		

Table 1. (Continued)

Variables	Normal child (N= 54)	Child with learning disability (N= 149)	Chi-square value	P
3	0 (0.0%)	1 (0.8%)		
Full term				
Yes	44 (97.8)	134 (94.4%)	0.87	0.35
No	1 (2.2%)	8 (5.6%)		
Type of delivery				
Vaginal	34 (72.3%)	86 (60.6%)	2.65	0.45
Surgery	11 (23.5%)	42 (29.6%)		
Assistance by equipment	1 (2.1%)	9 (6.3%)		
Induced by equipment	1 (2.1%)	5 (3.5%)		
Lack of oxygen in delivery				
Yes	5 (12.5%)	15 (11.9%)	0.01	0.92
No	35 (87.5%)	111 (88.1%)		
Age M(SD)	7.88 (1.18)	8.06 (1.78)	0.63	0.53
Size of Accommodation for each person in a family M(SD)	9.37 (9.03)	12.17 (17.36)	1.06	0.29
Birth weight M(SD)	3187.73 (460.31)	3289.73 (612.69)	1.02	0.31
Time length of lacking oxygen M(SD)	10.07 (16.74)	2.13 (2.10)	-1.56	0.15

There were more boys in the study group than control group, and more parents in the study groups used 'simple, rigid and autocratic', and 'inconsistent' education methods. In addition, there were more children in the study group living in apartments than those in the control group. There were no significant differences in child ages, disease history, birth status, parity, sleeping status, type of delivery, size of accommodation, birth weight, and time length of lack of oxygen. Table 2 demonstrates the difference between study and control groups in visual and auditory abilities. There were statistical significant differences between the two groups in auditory comprehension, visual memory, visual closure, and verbal expression, and also in total auditory and visual abilities scores. There were no differences between the two groups in auditory memory, auditory association and visual association, grammar, and manual expression. Table 3 presents results concerning associations among visual ability and auditory abilities in the study and control groups. The results show that the learning difficulty group showed a different correlation pattern from the normal children group. In the learning difficult group, five components of visual abilities and auditory abilities are significantly interrelated, and all visual ability components are significantly inter-correlated with auditory abilities components. In the normal children group, visual abilities are significantly inter-correlated. Most components of auditory abilities are significantly inter-correlated except the relationship between verbal expression to auditory reception, auditory association, and auditory working memory. Most components of visual abilities are statistically inter-correlated with components of auditory abilities with the exception of the relationship of visual memory and auditory reception, and the relationship of verbal expression to visual memory and visual closure.

Table 2. Comparison in visual and auditory abilities between children with learning difficulties and normal children

Variables	Normal child (n=50) M (S D)	Child with learning disability (n=149) M (S D)	t	P
Visual reception	37.67 (9.05)	39.77 (9.84)	1.34	0.18
Auditory reception	22.21 (6.96)	19.33 (6.62)	**2.66**	**0.008**
Visual memory	18.04 (5.31)	16.03 (7.62)	1.76	**0.008**
Auditory memory	35.89 (14.27)	35.40 (9.93)	0.27	0.79
Auditory Association	28.20 (8.33)	29.08 (8.29)	0.65	0.52
Visual Association	25.22 (8.52)	24.21 (9.07)	0.70	0.49
Visual Closure	34.79 (10.19)	29.46 (11.08)	**3.04**	**0.003**
Grammar	22.12 (5.94)	21.34 (8.17)	0.62	0.54
Manual expression	27.21 (4.57)	26.01 (6.79)	1.14	0.26
Verbal Expression	22.29 (6.26)	20.16 (6.41)	**2.06**	**0.04**
Total auditory ability	26.00 (6.00)	23.75 (4.99)	**2.58**	**0.01**
Total visual ability	28.52 (6.11)	25.51 (6.09)	**2.92**	**0.004**
Visual and auditory Memory	26.96 (8.10)	24.27 (6.23)	**2.45**	**0.02**
visual and auditory Closure	28.34 (7.45)	23.86 (7.90)	**3.48**	**0.001**
Visual and auditory association	26.60 (7.71)	25.18 (6.96)	1.21	0.23
Visual and auditory reception	29.83 (6.92)	28.12 (6.44)	1.60	0.11
Visual and auditory Expression	24.81 (4.25)	21.60 (4.76)	**4.14**	**0.001**

Table 3. Association between visual and auditory abilities

Groups	Abilities		1	2	3	4	5	6	7	8	9
Learning difficulties	1. visual reception:		1.00								
	2. Auditory reception	R	0.44	1.00							
		P	0.00								
	3. Visual memory	R	0.41	0.42	1.00						
		P	0.00	0.00							
	4. Auditory Association	R	0.50	0.55	0.61	1.00					
		P	0.00	0.00	0.00						
	5. Auditory memory	R	0.33	0.24	0.44	0.50	1.00				
		P	0.00	0.00	0.00	0.00					
	6. Visual Association	R	0.40	0.42	0.41	0.57	0.27	1.00			
		P	0.00	0.00	0.00	0.00	0.00				
	7. Visual Closure	R	0.52	0.46	0.53	0.63	0.40	0.50	1.00		
		P	0.00	0.00	0.00	0.00	0.00	0.00			
	8. Verbal Expression	R	0.55	0.48	0.56	0.62	0.31	0.48	0.49	1.00	
		P	0.00	0.00	0.00	0.00	0.00	0.00	0.00		
	9. grammar	R	0.57	0.52	0.60	0.72	0.48	0.56	0.61	0.62	1.00
		P	0.00	0.00	0.00	0.00	0.00	0.00	0.00	0.00	
	10. Manual expression	R	0.50	0.49	0.51	0.56	0.39	0.52	0.53	0.54	0.54
		P	0.00	0.00	0.00	0.00	0.00	0.00	0.00	0.00	0.00

Normal children	1. visual reception:		1.00								
	2. Auditory reception	R	**0.51**	1.00							
		P	0.00								
	3. Visual memory	R	**0.32**	0.23	1.00						
		P	0.02	0.11							
	4. Auditory Association	R	**0.51**	**0.47**	**0.49**	1.00					
		P	0.00	0.00	0.00						
	5. Auditory memory	R	**0.38**	**0.34**	0.20	**0.56**	1.00				
		P	0.01	0.01	0.15	0.00					
	6. Visual Association	R	**0.62**	**0.64**	**0.30**	**0.68**	**0.36**	1.00			
		P	0.00	0.00	0.03	0.00	0.01				
	7. Visual Closure	R	**0.49**	**0.54**	**0.54**	**0.78**	**0.52**	**0.65**	1.00		
		P	0.00	0.00	0.00	0.00	0.00	0.00			
	8. Verbal Expression	R	**0.33**	0.22	0.22	0.18	-0.16	**0.40**	0.16	1.00	
		P	0.02	0.11	0.11	0.20	0.27	0.00	0.26		
	9. grammar	R	**0.53**	**0.39**	**0.57**	**0.77**	**0.62**	**0.59**	**0.63**	**0.25**	1.00
		P	0.00	0.01	0.00	0.00	0.00	0.00	0.00	0.08	
	10. Manual expression	R	**0.69**	**0.53**	**0.33**	**0.61**	**0.50**	**0.55**	**0.61**	**0.24**	**0.61**
		P	0.00	0.00	0.02	0.00	0.00	0.00	0.00	0.10	0.00

Discussion

This study indicates that poor visual and auditory abilities are significantly related to learning difficulties, and parental education method and gender are also significant predictors of learning difficulties. The significant difference between the study and control groups in visual and auditory abilities, and significant associations between visual and auditory abilities in the study group suggest that children with learning difficulties may have problems processing information using their visual sensory and auditory sensory channels in a coordinated and integrative manner. These findings, which are consistent with published studies (1,2), may be due to children with learning difficulties lack coordination and integration of visual comprehension of written materials, visual-motor, visual processing, and visual working memory. (8). Children with learning difficulties also had additional deficits in auditory comprehension, and verbal expression of information.

It is noted that children with learning difficulties have lower scores in visual working memory but not in verbal working memory, suggesting that poor academic performance and information processing abilities may be related to subtle neurological development deficits in the brain. Spatial working memory ability is governed by the prefrontal lobe of the brain. Deficits in working memory in children with learning difficulties may indicate their poor development in specific abilities and these abilities are linked to problems with neurological development in the prefrontal lobe (3).

Children with learning difficulties in the present study did not have perinatal antecedents. All children in the study group had normal birth weight. They also did not differ from normal children in disease history, age, sleeping status, size of accommodation that they lived, and delivery type when they were born. The statistically significant difference between the learning difficulty and normal children groups in parental education method and living status suggest that 'simple, rigid and autocratic', 'inconsistent' education methods, and living in an apartment may restrict and limit the opportunities for them to develop sufficient self-esteem and confidence, and 'normal' visual spatial and auditory abilities (9).

The limitations of this study include the small number of children in the control group that may have led to a bias in results. The study was conducted in the clinical setting, which may limit the generalisability of the conclusions to the school community setting. Future studies should examine the interplay between visual-auditory abilities, family and school environment, and neurological characteristics, so intervention strategies can be developed that target groups of children with specific deficits and environments. It is recommended that the prevention of learning difficulties should focus on the development of adequate visual and auditory abilities including comprehension, perception, association and coordination, expression in school aged children. Health promotion programs should coordinate and promote both visual and auditory ability development in children at an early age to prevent deficits that impact subsequent academic performance.

References

[1] Girbau D, Schwartz RG. Phonological working memory in Spanish-English bilingual children with and without specific language impairment. J Commun Disord 2008;41(2):22.

[2] Torrioli MG, Frisone MF, Bonvini L, Luciano R, Pasca MG, Lepori R, et al. Perceptual-motor, visual and cognitive ability in very low birthweight preschool children without neonatal ultrasound abnormalities. Brain Dev 2000;22(3):163-8.

[3] Mammarella IC, Lucangeli D, Cornoldi C. Spatial working memory and arithmetic deficits in children with nonverbal learning difficulties. J Learn Disabil 2010;43(5):455-68.

[4] Menghini D, Carlesimo GA, Marotta L, Finzi A, Vicari S. Developmental dyslexia and explicit long-term memory. Dyslexia 2010;16(3):213-25.

[5] Goldstein DJ, Britt TW. Visual-motor coordination and intelligence as predictors of reading, mathematics, and written language ability. Percept Mot Skills 1994;78 (3 Pt 1):819-23.

[6] Belford B, Blumergh M. Factor analytic study of the revised Illinois test of Psycholinguistic Abilities (ITPA). Percept Mot Skills 1975;40:153-4.

[7] Kirk SA. Summaries of research on the revised Illinois Test of Psycliolinguistic Abilities. Tucson, AZ: University Arizona, 1972.

[8] Jongmans M, Mercuri E, de Vries L, Dubowitz L, Henderson SE. Minor neurological signs and perceptual-motor difficulties in prematurely born children. Arch Dis Child Fetal Neonatal Ed 1997;76(1):F9-14.

[9] Lahane S, Shah H, Nagarale V, Kamath R. Comparison of self-esteem and maternal attitude between children with learning disability and unaffected Siblings. Indian J Pediatr 2012 Nov 22.

In: Health Promotion
Editors: J. Sun, N. Buys, J. Merrick
ISBN: 978-1-62257-870-2

Chapter V

Relationship between resilience and quality of life in Chinese undergraduate university students

***Jing Sun, PhD**[*1] **and Nicholas Buys, PhD**[2]*
[1]School of Public Health and Griffith Health Institute, Griffith University, Gold Coast Campus, Parkland, Australia
[2]School of Human Services and Social Work, and Griffith Health Institute, Griffith University, Parkland, Gold Coast, Australia

Abstract

In this chapter we aim to investigate the relationship between resilience and quality of life (QOL) amongst undergraduate students across nine Beijing universities in China. A two stage cluster randomly selected sample and study design was used. There were 2,700 students were invited to attend to the study, and 2,046 students responded to the survey with high response rate of 75.8 percent. A standardised QOL questionnaire was used to assess university students perceived physical,

[*] *Correspondence:* Jing Sun, PhD, School of Public Health, Griffith University and Griffith Health Institute, Griffith University, Gold Coast Campus, Parkland, Q4222Australia. E-mail: j.sun@griffith.edu.au

mental health of QOL. Standardised resilience scales were used to determine their association with QOL. Multivariate linear regression analysis was used to analyse the association of QOL to resilience and social capital while demographic variables including age and gender were adjusted in the model. There were 26 percent of variances explained by resilience for physical health and 27.7 percent explained for mental health of QOL. The strongest explanatory variables in determining QOL were primarily focused on the individual's perception of self in the context of being a student (sense of self-acceptance, sense of autonomy, purpose of life, and personal growth) and also based on their involvement in the wider population (environmental mastery, and relations with others). These results suggest that resilience is an important factor to determine their QOL when they develop their ability to cope university life and be prepared to transit to the adult life.

Introduction

Quality of life (QOL) in undergraduate students has become an important clinical and community concern internationally (refs). QOL is most commonly construed as a multidimensional construct. The most commonly used definition of QOL is based on World Health Organization's (WHO's) definition of health including physical, mental components (1-3). QOL is defined by the WHOQOL Group (1994) as: "A person's perception of his / her position in life within the context of the culture and value systems in which they live, and in relation to their goals, expectations, standards, and concerns" (4). Poor QOL can result in poor academic performance and negative employment outcome.

University students face a range of stressors in their university life: for example, academic pressures, financial problems, and employment concerns. This can all affect their QOL. This situation is exemplified in Chinese university students as most undergraduate students are single children who are characterised as self-centered, with poor communication skills and capacity for self-regulation (5,6). Resilience has been found an important factor affecting QOL (1-3). Resilience is defined as the capacity of individuals, schools, families and communities to cope successfully with everyday challenges including life transitions, times of cumulative stress and significant adversity or risk. Typically, resilient individuals have high self-esteem, internal locus of control, optimism and clear aspirations, reflectiveness and problem solving capacity, respect for the autonomy of themselves and others, healthy communication patterns, and the capacity to seek out friends and environmental supports. These factors can prevent negative outcomes, as resilient individuals tend to have higher self-esteem, positive relations with others and an improved outlook on their life (7-9).

In China, the challenge has never been greater to raise children who are able to stand their ground amid growing educational, social and economic pressures, and increasing adolescent and youth mental disorders such as depression, eating disorders and other antisocial behaviours including drug abuse (10). The term the term "resilience" has been typically applied to youth who have overcome difficult situations such as abuse, neglect, poverty or school failure and gone on to become satisfied, productive and successful adults (5-7). But more recently, it has been recommended that schools, universities and educators can learn to help all youth to develop a "resilient mind-set."

Stress and adversity are an inevitable part of life in university students and therefore it makes sense to introduce resilience building strategies to youth in university. Resiliency promotion programs for youth have existed since the 1970's and have focused primarily on building self-esteem, increasing school readiness and supporting interpersonal relationships. Most promotion efforts, however, have tended to overlook the importance of multiple strategies that involve educational and social processes in the development of resilience, handling of stress and dealing with adversity to promote a good QOL. However, one of the neglected issues in research on QOL is adolescence, in particular among university youth in China. University youth is marked by biological, social role, and psychological changes, especially in rapid social and economic change times in China, and how they adapt to these changes can impact their transition into adulthood. If the additional stress of study impedes their development and successful transition, it is important to learn if this can be altered or buffered by promoting their resilience level. Despite the important role that resilience play in QOL in university students, there is limited research has explored the relationship between resilience and QOL in university students in China.

The primary hypothesis developed to guide this study framework was that a sense of resilience is significantly related to high level of QOL among Chinese university students'. It is postulated that positive scores in resilience will be significant indicators of QOL in the university. Deviations (i.e. negative or insignificant regression coefficients) from this trend in resilience would presumably result in a negative or insignificant impact on the QOL of university students. The aim of this study was therefore to determine the health-related QOL of university students, and how it is affected by the presence of resilience characteristics.

Our study

Two stage stratified randomly selected sampling was implemented at both university and individual student levels. There were nine university in Beijing from eligible 59 universities were randomly selected first then students were randomly selected from each of the nine universities. Survey method was used and a survey was administered during normal class hours. In total, 2,700 students were invited to take part in the study, and 2,046 students completed the survey with high response rate of 75.8%. The majority of students were freshmen and second year students. Written informed consent was obtained from the participating students. Ethical clearance was obtained from the human ethics committee at the Peking University, China.

Measures

Self-reported questionnaire were included in the survey instrument. These questionnaires include Chinese versions of the original standardised scales. Demographic characteristics included age, gender, place of origin, family income, and university year level.

Quality of Life measures: The World Health Organisation Quality of Life brief questionnaire (WHOQOL) was used to assess QOL in university students. For the purpose of this paper, two components of QOL were measured: physical and mental health. The WHOQOL-BREF is considered to be suitable for the current study because of its proven value as a cross-culturally valid and reliable instrument and its ease of completion with only 26 questions. A further advantage is that normative data are also available for the children population represented in the survey (with indications of sex differences and age trends), together with information of the scale of differences to be expected between 'well' people drawn from community settings and 'ill' people, with a wide range of existing health problems, drawn from health care contexts. Detailed normative data has recently been published by the Chinese WHOQOL group (11). The QOL scale has a good reliability with Cronbach Alpha level of more than 0.70 (12)

Respondents were asked to choose from four possible responses in a Likert format, where 1 is "very disatisfied" and 5 is "very satisfied". Scores range from 0 to 100 for each dimension of QOL after the scores were standardised, with higher scores reflecting greater levels of satisfaction of life. A score of less than 75 is suggestive of the lower than average score in either physical and mental health, as it was strongly associated with major depression (13).

Resilience: The resilience questionnaire developed by Ryff and Keyes (14) was used to measure six aspects of resilience. This includes: self-acceptance, the establishment of quality ties to others, a sense of autonomy in thought and action, the ability to manage complex environments to suit personal needs and values, the pursuit of meaningful goals and a sense of purpose in life, and continued growth and development as a person. The resilience questionnaire has six components that each component has 14 questions, and 84 questions in total. The scale uses a five-point Likert scale asking 1 is strongly disagree to 5 is strongly agree, and participants only need to select one answer among the five choices. A higher score indicates a higher level of resilience for each component. Resilience scale has good reliability and validity (14).

Statistical analysis

All data were analysed using SPSS package version 22.0. Descriptive statistics (means and standard deviations) of resilience and QOL scores are presented. Both bivariate (unadjusted) and multivariate (adjusted) linear regression was used to determine the possible relation of the explanatory variables, resilience and QOL in Chinese university students, the outcome variable. The confounding demographic information variables were used in the adjusted multivariate model to explain the significance of resilience on four main components physical health, psychological health, social functioning and environmental health of QOL.

Linear regression analyses using both bivariate and multivariate were performed for each QOL component. Confounding factors including age, gender, family socioeconomic status, university academic ranking, previous living condition, year of university were controlled in the analysis. Significance level was determined at $p < 0.05$ (2-tailed) for all multiple linear regression analyses.

Our findings

There were 2,700 students initially invited to participate in the study, with a final sample of 2,046, representing a high response rate of 75.8%. Of this sample 62.2% were males, 37.8% females, with ages ranging from 16 to 31 years old (*Mean age* = 19, SD = 1). Sixty-seven percent of the participants were first-year students, 18.5% second-year students, 11.0% third-year students and 3.2% fourth-year students (Table 2). Names of the university institution published in the website based on the Thompson Reuter index, with their ranking and stratified sample sizes (n) and percentage (%) are shown in Table 1 below. Equivalent sample sizes at both university rank, and within-university level was obtained.

Table 1. Nine Beijing universities of varying rank and number of sample sizes for each university

University ranking and number/percentage of students sampled	*n*	%
Excellent level		
1	288	14.1
2	195	9.5
3	179	8.7
Total	662	32.3
Good level		
1	283	13.8
2	239	11.7
3	184	9.0
Total	706	34.5
Average level		
1	216	10.6
2	244	11.9
3	218	10.7
Total	678	33.2

Information in regard to family background was also collected with 82% of individuals coming from two-parent households, and the average student living with 3-4 family members. Mean family income was 10,000-29,000 Chinese yuan and the geographical location of residence indicated a significant portion of students came from rural areas (43.7%), with 36.1% from the capital city, and 20.2% from other urban cities. Almost a quarter (24.1%) of individuals stated they had an existing health problem, but when asked of perceived health condition, 25.8% stated they were normal, 37.6% had good health and 34.6% believed they had very good or excellent health. Only 2.1% of respondents stated they had very poor health.

Table 2. Sample demographics at individual and family level with individual health perception of each participant

Variable	N (%)
University rank	
Top	662 (32.40)
Medium	706 (34.50)
Low	678 (33.10)
Family structure	
Double parents	1689 (82.60)
Single parent	357 (17.40)
Persons living together	
2	169 (8.30)
3	1043 (51.00)
4	611 (29.90)
5	174 (8.50)
6-11	49 (2.40)
Age group	
16-20 years	1760 (86.00)
21-30 years	286 (14.00)
Gender	
Male	1273 (62.20)
Female	773 (37.80)
Years in university	
1	578 (28.3)
2	478 (23.4)
3	425 (20.8)
4	565(27.6)
Income group	
Less than 10,000	586 (28.60)
10,000-29,999	830 (40.60)
30,333-59,999	353 (17.30)
60,000 and above	277 (13.50)
City living	
Capital city	738 (36.10)
Small city	413 (20.20)
Rural	895 (43.70)
Health status	
Very bad	43 (2.10)
Normal	527 (25.80)
Good	769 (37.60)
Very good	523 (25.60)
Excellent	184 (9.00)
Whether have health problem	
Yes	502 (24.5)
No	1544 (75.5)

Descriptive analysis result for QOL and resilience

Total scores of QOL and resilience were analysed using descriptive statistics prior to linear regression (see table 3). QOL total scores means ranged from 47.32 (physical health) to 49.38 (psychological health) within observed range = 0-100. Resilience mean values remained fairly constant in each resilience factor, ranging from 50.22 to 52.45. All resilience and QOL measure have normal distribution with skewness and kurtosis are within accepted range of -3 to +3.

Table 3. Descriptive statistics in QOL and resilience

	Mean	SD	Range	Skewness	Kurtosis
Quality of Life					
Physical Health	47.32	15.65	0-100	0.21	0.20
Psychological Health	49.38	16.30	0-100	0.21	-0.05
Resilience					
Autonomy	50.22	4.91	30-75	0.83	2.80
Environmental mastery	51.10	5.46	24-80	0.88	2.31
Personal growth	52.15	8.47	27-82	1.16	1.12
Positive relations	52.45	8.02	31-84	1.45	1.88
Purpose in life	51.47	5.83	24-80	1.00	2.96
Self-acceptance	50.98	5.65	28-77	1.12	2.28

Multiple linear regresslon results

Linear regression was implemented to identify the possible relationship that resilience had on four QOL factors: physical health, psychological health. Comparisons in statistical analysis were also made between unadjusted bivariate analysis and subsequent adjusted multivariate analysis to quantify the possible impact of demographic information into a QOL model.

Table 4 indicates that resilience significantly related to physical health of QOL. These effects are significant even when confounding factors including gender, university academic ranking, family structure, geographic living before they came to university, and health status.

Table 4. Linear regression for resilience and social capital (for QoL: physical health)

	Crude model			Adjusted model		
Variable	B (CI)	SE	*P* value	B (CI)	SE	*P* value
Resilience						
Autonomy	0.16 (0.03-0.29) *	0.07	0.02	0.17 (0.05-0.29) **	0.06	0.01
Environment mastery	0.53 (0.39-0.66) ***	0.07	<0.001	0.34 (0.21-0.46) ***	0.07	<0.001
Personal growth	0.29 (0.18-0.39) ***	0.05	<0.001	0.17 (0.08-0.27) ***	0.05	<0.001
Positive relations	0.30 (0.18-0.41) ***	0.06	<0.001	0.20 (0.09-0.30) ***	0.06	<0.001
Purpose in life	-0.10(-0.24-0.02)	0.07	0.05	-0.12 (-0.23-0.00)*	0.06	0.05
Self acceptance	0.31 (0.16-0.45) ***	0.07	<0.001	0.24 (0.11-0.38) ***	0.07	<0.001
University rank				-0.50 (-1.19-0.19)	0.35	0.15
Family structure				-1.75 (-3.35--0.15) *	0.82	0.03
Sex				0.69 (-0.48-1.86)	0.60	0.25
Years in university				-0.89 (-1.63--0.16)	0.38	0.02
City living				0.61 (-0.03-1.25)	0.33	0.06
Health condition				1.86 (1.27-2.46)	0.30	<0.001
Persons living together				-0.16 (-0.84-0.52)	0.35	0.65
Income group				-0.28 (-0.85-0.30)	0.29	0.344
	$R^2 = 24.10\%$, df = 6			$R^2 = 26.00\%$, df = 22		

* p<.05, ** p < 0.01, *** p < 0.001.

Table 5. Linear regression for resilience and social capital (for QoL: psychological health)

	Crude model			Adjusted model		
Variable	B (CI)	SE	*P* value	B (CI)	SE	*P* value
Resilience						
Autonomy	0.16 (0.02-0.30)*	0.07	0.02	0.16 (0.04-0.29)**	0.06	0.01
Environmental mastery	0.49 (0.35-0.64)***	0.07	<0.001	0.28 (0.14-0.41)***	0.07	<0.001
Personal growth	0.19 (0.08-0.29)***	0.05	<0.001	0.08(-0.01-0.18)*	0.05	0.04
Positive relations	0.21 (0.10-0.33)***	0.06	<0.001	0.12(0.01-0.23)*	0.06	0.03
Purpose in life	0.31 (0.18-0.44)***	0.07	<0.001	0.31 (0.18-0.43)***	0.06	<0.001
Self acceptance	0.43 (0.28-0.58)***	0.08	<0.001	0.38 (0.24-0.52)***	0.07	<0.001
University rank				-0.17(-0.88-0.54)	0.36	0.63
Family structure				0.01(-1.64-1.66)	0.84	0.99
Sex				0.28(-0.92-1.49)	0.61	0.65
Years in university				-0.88(-1.64-0.12)*	0.39	0.02
City living				-0.38(-1.04-0.28)	0.34	0.26
Health condition				1.39(0.77-2.00)***	0.31	<0.001
Persons living together				0.13(-0.57-0.83)	0.36	0.72
Income group				0.46(-0.14-1.05)	0.30	0.13
	R^2 = 26.70%, df = 6			R^2 = 27.7%, df = 22		

* p<.05, ** p < 0.01, *** p < 0.001.

Discussion

This study investigated the relationship between resilience and QOL. All possible confounding factors, demographics, was investigated in an adjusted multivariate model and compared with the original crude bivariate model. Results indicate a positive and significant correlation between QOL and the resilience in both crude unadjusted and multivariate adjusted models, thus supporting the original hypothesis. In this study 24% of the sample reported a number of physical health problems, a substantial number that is of concern as low resilience can exacerbate physical health problems.

Resilience has a significantly positive relationship with physical health of QOL even when confounding factors were controlled in the multiple regression model. The six components of resilience scale were all significantly related to physical health of QOL. The relationship between self-acceptance and physical health indicates that with an increasing level of self-acceptance there is an increasing level of positive attitude towards self-appearance, positive feelings and confidence in managing physical health. The finding of an association between positive relations with others and physical health suggests that the presence of warm, satisfying and trusting relationships with self and others assists in dealing with physical health issues. Sense of autonomy is related to physical health, indicating that individuals rating high on this characteristic are able to self-determine and independently deal with bodily pain and disease issues. The relationship between environmental mastery and physical health suggests that with an increasing level of sense of mastery individuals are able to manage environmental support, and control resources when they deal with any physical illness. The relationship between sense of directedness and physical health indicates the beliefs that give life meaning are important for university students to deal with and manage physical health towards positive development. The relationship between personal growth and physical health suggests that having a sense of improvement or expansion over time, and feels interested in life encourages students to actively s to manage and control their physical health.

The significant relationship between all components of resilience and mental health suggest that resilience is predictive of mental health status of university students. This is consistent with the findings of previous research, low level of resilience can contribute to psychological distress and depression (15). Our findings also indicate that personal level characteristics such as sense of self-acceptance, sense of autonomy, purpose of life personal growth, and environmental related characteristics such as environmental mastery and relations with other were associated with mental health status. This is because decreasing levels of resilience decrease the opportunities to develop individual self-esteem and coping strategies through external supports, and, more importantly, hinders the capacity of the individual to buffer and cope stressful situations (16,17).

The study has two limitations. First, the study is a cross-sectional study so the interpretation of the causal relationship between resilience and QOL need to be treated with cautioun. Second, the study used the self-reported measure to assess QOL so the results may be viewed as subjective. Further research should be conducted to include other settings and cities in China as there may be differences between students in metropolitan Beijing and students at universities located in rural and remote areas. A prospective study design is recommended for the next stage of the study to determine the causal relationship between resilience and QoL, and more objective measures such as anthropometry and biomedical methods used to measure physical and mental health status of the university students.

In conclusion, resilience has been found significantly related to physical and mental health in university students. It is recommended that university health promotion policies and activities focus on the development programs to enhance resilience of university students to prevent the development of physical and mental health problems and thereby facilitate students' academic work and successful transition to adult life.

References

[1] Drukker M, Kaplan C, Feron F, Os JV. Children's health-related quality of life, neighborhood socio-economic deprivation and social capital. A contextual analysis. Soc Sci Med 2003;57:825-41.

[2] Jirojanakul P, Skevington SM, Hudson J. Predicting young children's quality of life. Soc Sci Med 2003;57:1277-88.

[3] Lawford J, Eiser C. Exploring links between the concepts of Quality of Life and Resilience. Pediatr Rehabil 2001;4(1):209-16.

[4] WHOQOL Group. Thg World Health Organization quality of life assessment (WHOQOL): Development and general psyhcometric propterties. Soc Sci Med 1998;46(12):1569-85.

[5] Sun J, Stewart D. Age and gender effects on resilience in children and adolescents.Pediatr Rehabil 2007;9(4):16-25.

[6] Sun J, Stewart D, Yuan BJ, Zhang SH. Validation of General Health Questionnaire-30 in parents with primary school children. Compr Psychiatry 2011, in press.

[7] Masten A, Best KM, Garmezy N. Resiliency and development: Contributions from the study of children who overcome adversity. Dev Psychopathol 1991;2:425-44.

[8] Rutter M. Psychosocial resilience and protective mechanisms. In: Rolf J, Masten A, Cicchetti D, Nuechterlein K, Weintraub S, eds. Risk and protective factors in the development of psychopathology. New York: Cambridge University Press, 1990.

[9] Sun J, Stewart D. Development of population based resilience measures in the primary school setting. Health Educ 2007;107(6):575-99.

[10] Sun J, Buys N, Wang XC. Depressive symptoms, family Functioning, university environment, and social support: a population based study in university students in Beijing China. Int J Psychol Behav Sci 2011;1(1):41-7.

[11] Skevington SM, Lotfy M, O'Connell KA, Group W. The World Health Organization's WHOQOL-BREF quality of life assessment: psychometric properties and results of the international field trial. A report from the WHOQOL group. Qual Life Res 2004;13(2):299-310.

[12] WHO. WHOQoL-OLD. Geneva: World Health Organization, 2006.

[13] Kroenke K, Outcalt S, Krebs E, Bair MJ, Wu J, Chumbler N, et al. Association between anxiety, health-related quality of life and functional impairment in primary care patients with chronic pain. Gen Hosp Psychiatry 2013, in press.

[14] Ryff C, Keyes C. The structure of psychological well-being revisited. J Pers Soc Psychol 1995;69:719-27.

[15] Gerber M, Kalak N, Lemola S, Clough PJ, Perry JL, Pühse U, et al. Are adolescents with high mental toughness levels more resilient against stress? Stress Health 2013;29(2):164-71.

[16] Jia-Yan P. A resilience-based and meaning-oriented model of acculturation: A sample of mainland Chinese postgraduate students in Hong Kong. Int J Intercult Relat 2011;35(5):592-603.

[17] Malti T, Noam GG. The hidden crisis in mental health and education: the gap between student needs and existing supports. New Dir Youth Dev 2008(120):13-29.

In: Health Promotion
Editors: J. Sun, N. Buys, J. Merrick

ISBN: 978-1-62257-870-2

Chapter VI

Validation of shared decision-making questionnaire in the dental encounter

Jessica Peters, BA, BOralH[1], Florian Mack, PhD[1] and Jing Sun, PhD[2*]

[1]School of Oral Health and Dental Science, Griffith University, Centre for Medicine and Oral Health, Southport, Australia
[2]School of Public Health and Griffith Health Institute, Griffith University, Logan campus, Meadowbrook, Australia

Abstract

Communication within the dental encounter is paramount to successful clinical outcomes. In this chapter we examine the concept of shared decision-making (SDM) in patients who have received treatment for a single missing tooth. Method: A cross sectional study design was used for the study. Patients were recruited from a university dental clinic and a private dental practice. Exploratory factor analysis was used to identify the dimensions of patient's SDM, their level of dental knowledge and

* *Correspondence:* Jing Sun, PhD, School of Public Health, Griffith University and Griffith Health Institute, Griffith University, Gold Coast Campus, Parkland, Q4222 Australia. E-mail: j.sun@griffith.edu.au.

their treatment satisfaction. Results: Exploratory factor analysis showed that 9 factors were extracted from the questionnaire. Overall, the 9 factor structure had a high level of reliability for each individual dimension. Of the 108 participants, only 26.5% were exposed to SDM. Independent sample t tests showed that there was no significant difference between the SDM group and comparison group on levels of denture knowledge, post treatment functional and economic satisfaction. However, a significant difference was seen in regards to knowledge of other treatment alternatives and post treatment aesthetic/social satisfaction, with the SDM group reporting higher levels. Conclusions: The results suggest that a 9 factor solution can be used to assess the patient's experience in the dental encounter. In regards to the use of SDM in the dental encounter, further research is required using a larger sample size from an increased number of dental practices. However, SDM is an important component of clinical dental practice and should be further explored in clinical dentistry.

Introduction

Patient participation in medical decision-making is receiving increasing emphasis (1). Over the decades there has been a profound change in the clinician patient relationship (2). This change is represented by a shift from the paternalistic model (doctor decides, patient complies without any explanations) to the informative model (doctor provides information, patient decides) (1,3). This paradigm shift has resulted in an increased focus on shared decision-making between doctors and patients. The informative model gives patients the opportunity to participate in decisions by expressing his or her preferences among alternative treatment options (2). When selecting a treatment for a specific medical condition, there is rarely one treatment that is clearly superior to others (1). Given the variety of treatment options for most medical problems, the responsibility for choosing a treatment should be shared by both the clinician and the patient and thus a shared decision making (SDM) process should be employed (1).

SDM is defined as an approach in which the clinician and patient go through all phases of the decision making process together (1). SDM transcends the legal obligation of informed consent, which does not necessarily involve the shared discussion of treatment options, benefits and risks (4). When SDM is employed, information is provided about the health problem, the possible treatment options and consequences of the treatments are discussed, and together the clinician and patient consider how these fit with the patients preferred outcomes (1). After the options are considered, a treatment decision is made based on mutual agreement (5).

In order for SDM to be successfully achieved, certain criteria need to be obtained (5). Firstly, the doctor needs to provide an environment in the consultation where patient participation is encouraged and patients must feel that their contributions are valued (1). The goals of the patient and their desired treatment outcome must be discussed in the consultation (5). Individual patients vary in their preferences for health states, tolerances for pain and discomfort and future needs (5). Obtaining this information from the patient is crucial to selecting the most appropriate treatment option for an individual patient (5). Finally a critical characteristic of SDM is to provide the patients with sufficient information, including treatment alternatives and their possible consequences (6). This is to ensure that the patient is not making a decision in the face of avoidable ignorance (7).

Elwyn et al. (7) developed a three stage model of SDM that can act as a guide to skill development in routine clinical practice. The first stage, *introducing choice,* is to inform patients that options exist. The second stage, *option talk*, involves exploring the patient's existing knowledge, clarifying any incorrect knowledge that the patient may have and clearly outlining the pros and cons of the alternative treatment options (7). The final stage of the model is *decision talk*, which explores the need to either defer a decision or make an immediate decision (7). Allowing time for this is a cornerstone for effective SDM because patients often need to take the time to discuss their options with others in a form of deliberation process (7-9).

The concept of SDM has been thoroughly explored in clinical medicine. Numerous studies have reported improvements in patient satisfaction, treatment adherence, quality of life, and well-being when patients are more involved in their treatment choice (5,6,10-12). Similar to medicine, many dental problems have a variety of treatment options. It therefore follows that the responsibility for choosing the most suitable treatment should be shared by both the dentist and the patient thereby employing the SDM approach. However, little research on SDM was found in the dental literature. Therefore, an aim of this study was to examine whether dental professionals are engaging in SDM with their patients. While the concept of SDM has little presence in the dental literature, studies have sought to determine what the patient values in the dental encounter. It is evident that patients are less concerned with the technical competency of the dentist (13). Rather, patients view the communication skills of the dentist as most important (13, 14). For example, a study completed by Sbaraini et al (13) examined patient's experiences of dental care in Australia. They concluded that patients want a dentist who is caring and supportive, who listens to their concerns and takes time to explain treatment options and procedures. Patient's valued dentists who made them aware of the options, educated them about how to maintain a healthy mouth, and supported and reassured them frequently during visits (13). Research has also examined the factors that predict patient satisfaction after the dental encounter. Factors identified include; cost, convenience, technical competence with the largest factor being interpersonal skills of the dentist (14). This is consistent with literature from the medical field indicating that the most important predictor of patient satisfaction is the quality of the doctor-patient relationship (2,4,15). With the most important predictor of patient satisfaction being the ability of the dentist to communicate, it is postulated that dental patients would value SDM in the dental encounter. It is proposed that the use of SDM in the dental encounter is an effective way to enhance dental knowledge in dental patients and to achieve a high level of post treatment satisfaction among dental patients. In the medical literature, it has been argued that SDM is especially applicable to long-term health decisions and when the intervention requires more than one session (6). Many dental procedures fit these criteria, for instance, the treatment of missing teeth. The three key treatment modalities available for the replacement of missing teeth include; removable partial denture (RPD), fixed partial denture (FPD) and implant supported crown (16). There are both advantages and disadvantages associated with each treatment modality and this is well outlined within the literature (17). No matter which treatment option is selected, several appointments are required and the final choice will have a long-term impact on the patient. The purpose of this study was to develop a questionnaire to examine SDM in patients who have received dental treatment for a single missing tooth, with two specific aims in mind. Firstly, this chapter aims to determine if patients who have experienced SDM will have a higher level of knowledge of the treatment alternatives. Secondly, this study attempts to determine if patients who have experienced SDM will have a greater sense of treatment satisfaction.

Our study

A cross sectional study design was used to collect data from dental patients who either visited the Griffith University dental clinic or a private dental practice in Tasmania. Data was collected in December 2012 to February 2013.

Participants

Participants used in this study were patients who had received treatment for a single tooth gap. A single tooth gap is defined as a gap resulting from a single missing tooth that is bordered by one or more natural teeth on either side (18). Participants may have had multiple missing teeth, however the presence of a single tooth gap was required. Two inclusion criteria were used when selecting participants for this study. Participants must have received treatment for a single missing tooth and the treatment must have already been completed. Participants were selected from either the Griffith University dental clinic in Queensland or a private dental practice in Tasmania. Patients who had received this type of treatment were identified using computer records. The total sample comprised 109 patients; all whom had either received a removable partial denture, fixed partial denture or implant supported crown to replace their missing tooth. Ethics approval was obtained from the Griffith University Human Research Ethics Committee (reference no. D0H/27/12/HREC). Edentulous patients (patients will all their teeth missing), patients with no missing teeth, patients with missing wisdom teeth only and patients with multiple missing teeth in a row, were excluded from the study.

Research tools

A questionnaire was developed by the researchers to assess the patient's overall treatment experience. The questionnaire included 107 items that examined the patient's dental habits and history, the number of missing teeth prior to treatment, the types of treatment modalities discussed with them, the patient's knowledge of treatment alternatives, the recommendations provided by the dentist, and the final treatment choice.

Post treatment satisfaction was assessed on four different levels including; functional, aesthetic, social and economic satisfaction following dental treatment. Items were scored on a 2 point scale (1, yes; 0, no) or on a 6 point scale (5, strongly agree; 4, agree; 3, somewhat agree; 2, somewhat disagree; 1, disagree; 0, strongly disagree). The knowledge questions were scored based on a semantic scale ranging from 1 to 7.

Exposure to SDM was assessed by examining whether treatment alternatives were provided to the patient. Patients who were presented with all three treatment modalities were assigned to the SDM group. If the patient was only given two treatment options or simply told what treatment was best without exploring alternatives, it was assumed that SDM was not utilized and these patients were assigned to the comparison group. Demographic factors were also collated including; age, gender, income, place of residence, level of education, family and general health status. Information regarding whether or not the patient's treatment was covered by private health insurance or whether or not the patient received government assistance for their dental treatment was also collated.

Data collection

Patients who had received treatment for a single tooth gap were approached in both the private dental practice and the university dental clinic. These participants were provided with an information sheet outlining the purpose of the study and the study procedure.

Statistical analysis

Data analysis was completed using SPSS version 21.0. Statistical analysis was conducted on unweighted data. A principle component analysis was conducted to investigate the subscales structure within the questionnaire. Varimax rotation was considered appropriate for the current study, which uses an orthogonal rotation method that minimizes the number of variables that has high loadings on each factor. Exploratory factor analysis was used to extract the factor structure of the questionnairc. Pearsons correlation bivariate analysis was completed to ensure each factor was not highly correlated and represented an independent factor. Reliability was assessed from analyses of internal consistency using Cronbach α. Independent *t* tests were conducted to examine differences in satisfaction and knowledge between the SDM group and the comparison group.

Exploratory factor analysis

Exploratory factor analysis for the developed questionnaire was undertaken. The results are presented in table 1. Further analysis using the Scree test showed that nine factors could be meaningfully extracted (see figure 1). This nine factor solution can be considered as a relatively adequate representation of the data.

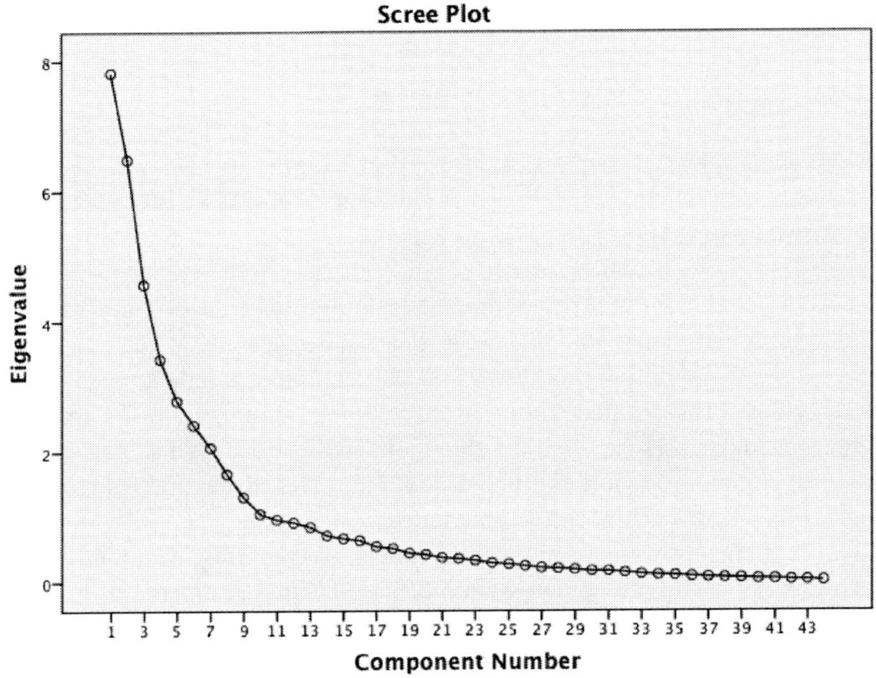

Figure 1. Nine factor extraction Scree plot based on factor analysis.

Our findings

One hundred-nine participants completed the survey with 100% response rate. Of these participants, 48.6% were aged between 45-64 years, while 45.9% were aged 65 years and above and only 5.5 % aged between 25-44 years. Among the respondents, 65 (59.6%) were female. Education levels indicated that 39.4 % had tertiary education, 14.7 % had diploma/Training and Further Education, 44.0 % had secondary education and only 1.8 % had primary education level. When looking at place of residence, 82 (75.9%) were from metropolitan/city area, 21 (19.4%) from a semi rural area and 5 (4.6%) from a rural area. In terms of family status, 84 (77.1%) were living in a relationship/partnership and 25 (22.9%) were single. When look at average household income, 32% of participants reported earning $37,000 or less,

34.9% reported $37,001-$80,000, 28.3% reported $80,001-$180,000, and 4.7% reported $180,001 and over per year. Although, 109 participants completed the survey, 106 participants answered all 107 items.

Dental characteristics of participants

Seventy-nine (72.5%) participants received private health insurance for their dental treatment whereas 21 (19.3%) received government assistance for their dental treatment. Eighteen (16.3%) participants from the total sample reported that they had previously been treated for gum disease. In regards to the number of missing teeth, 38 (34.9%) had only 1 missing tooth, 26 (24.1%) had 2-3 missing teeth and 45 (41.7%) had more than 3 missing teeth. When looking at the location of the missing tooth, 69 (63.3%) participants indicated that their missing tooth was located at the front of their mouth, with 74 (67.9%) participants indicating that their missing tooth could be seen when they smiled. The most commonly reported cause of tooth loss was; decay (35.8%), trauma (26.6%), cracked tooth (17.4%) and failed dental treatment (16.5%). Eight (7.3%) participants were unsure of the cause of their missing tooth. When looking at how long the patient waited before seeking treatment, 70 (64.2%) sought treatment immediately, 9 (8.3%) sought treatment within one year, 11 (10.1%) sought treatment within 1-3 years and, 19 (17.4%) waited more than 3 years for treatment. Finally, when looking at the final treatment choice, 41 (37.6%) participants received a fixed dental prosthesis, 32 (29.4%) participants received a chrome cobalt denture, 11 (10.1%) participants received an acrylic denture, and 27 (24.8%) participants received an implant retained crown.

Grouping of participants

Whether or not alternative treatment options were discussed with patients by their dentist was examined. It was found that only 29 (26.6%) participants were presented with all three treatment options and could subsequently be assigned to the SDM group. Twenty-one (19.3%) participants were presented with two treatment options, 57 (52.3%) participants were presented with one treatment option and two (1.8%) were not presented with any treatment options. These participants were assigned to the comparison group.

Factor analysis

The Exploratory Factor Analysis derived a nine component solution from the factor analysis (see table 1). Factor 1 [items 79, 93, 94, 95, 96, 97, 98] indicated the respondent's level of post treatment aesthetic and social satisfaction. For example: after the replacement of my missing tooth; I feel more confident, I am happier with how my mouth looks, and I feel more comfortable smiling. Factor 2 was knowledge of the two other treatment modalities; implant retained crown and FPD. This was assessed using items 66, 67, 68, 69, 70, and 71. Pre-treatment self esteem was the third factor, which included 6 items 84, 85, 86, 87, 88 and 89. For example; before my treatment I did not like meeting new people, I felt that people were staring at my missing tooth, I lacked confidence and I did not feel good about myself. Factor 4 represented the degree in which procedural factors impacted on the patient's treatment choice. This was measured using items 72, 73, 74, 75, 76, 77, and 78. The fifth factor comprised the oral health beliefs of the patient. This was measured using 5 items 101, 102, 103, 105, and 106 such as: I believe that; good teeth are important for general health, maintaining nutrition, and eating and chewing. Factor 6 included items 81, 82, and 83, which measured pretreatment masticatory functioning. Factor 7 included 3 items, which measured patient's satisfaction with post treatment masticatory functioning [items 90, 91, 92]. The eighth factor expressed the patient's level of denture knowledge, which was assessed using items 63, 64, and 65. The ninth and final factor was post treatment economic satisfaction. This was measured using item 99 and 100. Pearsons correlation bivariate analysis was completed to ensure each factor was not highly correlated (correlation < .85) and therefore represented an independent concept (see table 2).

All of the nine factors identified were normally distributed except for post treatment functional satisfaction. Therefore, non-parametric tests were applied to the analysis of this factor. The variance explained for the nine factors were 11.73%, 11.57%, 11.03%, 8.43%, 7.58%, 6.92%, 6.45%, 6.20%, and 4.02% respectively. The total variance explained by the nine factors was 73.93%.

Table 1. Principle component analysis for nine factor structure

	Post treatment aesthetic/ social satisfaction	Knowledge of other treatment modalities	Pre-treatment self esteem	Procedural factors	Oral health beliefs	Pre-treatment functioning	Post treatment functional satisfaction	Denture knowledge	Post treatment economic satisfaction
95. After the replacement of my missing tooth I am happier with how my mouth looks.	**.873**	-.007	.057	-.071	.162	-.040	.031	-.033	-.013
94. After the replacement of my missing tooth I feel more confident.	**.872**	.039	.143	.054	.198	.017	.092	-.068	.083
99. After the replacement of my missing tooth I feel more comfortable smiling.	**.855**	.097	.121	-.074	.189	-.059	.008	.019	.097
97. After the replacement of my missing tooth I now enjoy meeting new people.	**.808**	.092	.269	.050	.028	-.096	.159	.131	.067
96. After the replacement of my missing tooth I feel better about myself.	**.800**	.069	.111	.056	.076	.044	.176	.025	.203

	Post treatment aesthetic/ social satisfaction	Knowledge of other treatment modalities	Pre-treatment self esteem	Procedural factors	Oral health beliefs	Pre-treatment functioning	Post treatment functional satisfaction	Denture knowledge	Post treatment economic satisfaction
98. After the replacement of my missing tooth I now enjoy speaking in public.	**.735**	.170	.299	.044	-.006	-.126	.152	.182	.044
80. A major reason for the replacement of my missing tooth was my appearance.	**.441**	-.020	.302	-.086	.213	-.104	.030	.075	-.342
71. Did you know how an implant was inserted before your treatment?	.109	**.895**	-.017	-.102	.053	.138	-.067	.072	-.122
70. Did you know what an implant looked like before your treatment?	.030	**.885**	-.137	.030	.073	-.186	.152	.081	.115
72. Did you know how to clean an implant before your treatment?	.100	**.878**	-.031	-.116	.047	.169	-.005	.036	-.149
68. Did you know how a bridge was constructed before your treatment?	.125	**.874**	.012	-.079	.033	.183	-.089	.092	.002
69. Did you know how to clean a bridge before your treatment?	.045	**.852**	-.119	.050	.106	-.102	.132	.065	.068

Table 1. (Continued)

	Post treatment aesthetic/ social satisfaction	Knowledge of other treatment modalities	Pre-treatment self esteem	Procedural factors	Oral health beliefs	Pre-treatment functioning	Post treatment functional satisfaction	Denture knowledge	Post treatment economic satisfaction
67. Did you know what a bridge looked like before your treatment?	.022	**.805**	-.161	.016	.088	-.185	.189	.161	.045
73. Damage to the surrounding teeth through drilling was a factor that influenced my final treatment choice.	-.058	**.451**	.210	.420	.015	.142	-.026	.096	.143
88. Before my treatment I did not like meeting new people.	.135	-.099	**.886**	.188	-.057	.031	.032	.057	.014
90. Before my treatment I felt that people were staring at my missing tooth.	.232	.034	**.860**	.107	-.094	.041	-.074	.005	.014
86. Before my treatment I did not feel good about myself.	.116	-.032	**.854**	.108	.032	.168	.042	-.137	.101
85. Before my treatment I lacked confidence.	.088	-.109	**.854**	.162	-.061	.064	-.011	.114	.013

	Post treatment aesthetic/ social satisfaction	Knowledge of other treatment modalities	Pre-treatment self esteem	Procedural factors	Oral health beliefs	Pre-treatment functioning	Post treatment functional satisfaction	Denture knowledge	Post treatment economic satisfaction
89. Before my treatment I did not like speaking in public.	.099	-.056	**.852**	.174	.079	.148	.043	-.089	-.012
87. Before my treatment I was unhappy with how my mouth looked.	.312	-.129	**.701**	.021	.047	.141	-.055	.078	-.133
77. The amount of pain I associated with each procedure influenced my final treatment choice.	-.017	-.099	.141	**.875**	.024	.058	.063	-.023	.010
76. I experience fear/anxiety towards dental treatment and this influenced my final treatment choice.	.032	-.117	.019	**.806**	.069	.133	.023	.025	-.014
78. The amount of discomfort I associated with each procedure influenced my final treatment choice.	-.003	-.176	.100	**.800**	.041	.126	-.021	.039	-.065
74. Duration of the treatment was a factor that influenced my final treatment choice.	-.041	.159	.218	**.650**	-.251	.013	.043	-.015	.091

Table 1. (Continued)

	Post treatment aesthetic/ social satisfaction	Knowledge of other treatment modalities	Pre-treatment self esteem	Procedural factors	Oral health beliefs	Pre-treatment functioning	Post treatment functional satisfaction	Denture knowledge	Post treatment economic satisfaction
79. The materials that are used in each procedure were a factor that influenced my final treatment choice.	-.090	-.016	.001	**.612**	-.208	.041	-.161	-.018	-.301
75. Cost of the treatment was a factor that influenced my final treatment choice.	.112	.120	.202	**.612**	.035	.042	-.129	-.024	-.027
104. I believe that good teeth are important for my general health.	.158	.069	-.112	-.039	**.846**	-.015	.152	.090	.035
106. I believe that good teeth are important for eating and chewing.	.022	.094	-.059	-.083	**.781**	.055	.065	.059	.085
103. I believe that someone with all their teeth looks better than someone with missing teeth.	.020	.025	.087	-.089	**.764**	-.077	.074	.106	-.031

	Post treatment aesthetic/ social satisfaction	Knowledge of other treatment modalities	Pre-treatment self esteem	Procedural factors	Oral health beliefs	Pre-treatment functioning	Post treatment functional satisfaction	Denture knowledge	Post treatment economic satisfaction
107. I believe good teeth are important for maintaining nutrition.	.228	.132	-.018	.076	**.673**	.008	-.053	.074	.054
102. I believe that good teeth are important for my appearance	.412	-.030	.104	.044	**.648**	-.216	-.032	.085	-.034
105. I believe that missing or decayed teeth are a sign of poor health.	.352	.255	-.050	-.007	**.360**	.176	-.120	.050	.227
84. Before my treatment I found it difficult to eat crunchy vegetables.	.023	.058	.139	.169	-.046	**.882**	.128	-.036	-.008
82. Before my treatment I found it difficult to eat crunchy fruit.	.004	-.002	.182	.110	-.010	**.878**	.175	.026	-.065
83. Before my treatment I found it difficult to eat cooked meat.	-.139	.004	.183	.186	-.092	**.846**	.151	.051	.039
81. A major reason for the replacement of my missing tooth was my ability to eat and chew.	-.239	.042	.023	.014	.023	**.468**	.278	-.062	-.214
91. After the replacement of my missing tooth I can now eat crunchy fruit.	.118	.048	-.001	-.057	.030	.191	**.903**	-.035	.095

Table 1. (Continued)

	Post treatment aesthetic/ social satisfaction	Knowledge of other treatment modalities	Pre-treatment self esteem	Procedural factors	Oral health beliefs	Pre-treatment functioning	Post treatment functional satisfaction	Denture knowledge	Post treatment economic satisfaction
93. After the replacement of my missing tooth I can now eat crunchy vegetables.	.184	.120	.001	-.078	.067	.177	**.900**	-.006	.107
92. After the replacement of my missing tooth I can now eat cooked meat.	.193	.053	-.015	-.018	.101	.216	**.858**	.071	.105
66. Did you know how to clean a denture before your treatment?	.039	.119	.040	.033	.099	.021	-.010	**.929**	.116
65. Did you know how to use a denture before your treatment?	.028	208	-.022	.004	.126	.012	.057	**.926**	-.010
64. Did you know what a denture looked like before your treatment?	.116	.115	.008	-.020	.167	-.033	-.027	**.878**	-.057
101. I believe that I paid too much for my treatment (reversed).	.102	-.080	.021	-.133	.026	-.044	.146	-.021	**.786**
100. I believe that I received value for the cost of my dental treatment.	.232	.070	.027	-.019	.135	-.114	.113	.079	**.771**

Table 2. Inter-correlation between the nine factors obtained from factor analysis

	Post treatment physical and social satisfaction	Post treatment functional satisfaction	Post treatment economic satisfaction	Denture knowledge	Knowledge of other treatment modalities	Pre-treatment self esteem	Pre-treatment functioning	Procedural factors	Oral health beliefs
Post treatment physical and social satisfaction									
Post treatment functional satisfaction	.248*								
Post treatment economic satisfaction	.212*	.177							
Denture knowledge	.185	.020	.084						
Knowledge of other treatment modalities	.160	.085	0.26	.276**					
Pre-treatment self esteem	.408**	.063	.019	-.007	-.151				
Pre-treatment functioning	-.029	.230*	-.059	.011	.029	.284**			
Procedural factors	.056	-.046	-.149	.056	-.003	.305**	.263**		
Oral health beliefs	.400**	.097	.215*	.235*	.173	.052	-.089	-.094	

** Correlation is significant at the 0.01 level (2-tailed).

Reliability

The overall reliability level of the questionnaire was relatively high with a Cronbach α level of .86. Table 3 indicates that the subscales based on the 9 extracted factors were generally found to be reliable with levels ranging from .67 to .95.

Table 3. Reliability correlations, Cronbach α

Questionnaire	Reliability correlations, Cronbach *α* (9 factors)
Total score	.86
Post treatment aesthetic/social satisfaction	.92
Post treatment functional satisfaction	.95
Post treatment economic satisfaction	.67
Denture knowledge	.93
Knowledge of other treatment modalities	.95
Pretreatment self esteem	.93
Pretreatment functioning	.86
Procedural factors	.82
Oral health beliefs	.77

Discriminant validity of SDM questionnaire

An independent sample t-test was conducted to compare the SDM group and the comparison group on knowledge of treatment alternatives and treatment satisfaction (see table 4). In regards to denture knowledge, there was no significant difference between the two groups (*p* value .918). There was however a significant difference between the SDM group and the comparison group on level of knowledge of other treatment modalities (*p* value .020), with the SDM group showing a higher level of knowledge. When looking at treatment satisfaction, no significant difference was found between the SDM group and the comparison group on levels of post treatment functional satisfaction (*p* value .842 see table 5) or post treatment economic satisfaction (*p* value .755). There was however a significant difference between the SDM group and the comparison group on levels of post treatment aesthetic/social satisfaction (*p* value .031) with the SDM showing a higher level of satisfaction.

Table 4. Differences in dental knowledge and treatment satisfaction between the SDM group and the comparison group

Variables	Group		*t*	P value
	SDM group (n= 29) Mean (SD)	Comparison group (n= 79) Mean (SD)		
Knowledge				
Denture knowledge	15.03 (6.17)	15.18 (6.89)	-.103	.918
Knowledge of other treatment modalities	22.09 (13.67)	15.94 (12.13)	2.41	.020
Satisfaction				
Post treatment aesthetic/social satisfaction	26.28 (7.12)	22.47 (9.91)	2.20	.031
Post treatment economic satisfaction	6.97 (2.06)	7.12 (2.52)	-.314	.755

Table 5. Differences in post treatment functional satisfaction

Group	Median	Min, Max	Z score	P value
SDM group	12.00	.00, 15.00	-.200	.842
Comparison group	13.00	.00,15.00		

Discussion

Exploratory factor analysis in the current study showed a nine factor solution. A process was undertaken in order to reach the conclusion that nine factors were required. For the first factor analysis model, factor loading of less than 0.4 were suppressed and 10 factors were extracted based on Eigenvalue more than one. For the second factor analysis model, nine factors were selected. In comparison to the first model, the nine factors generated from the second factor analysis, better reflected the meaning of clustered questions. In the nine factor analysis item 72 and 101 cross loaded on two factors. These items were subsequently placed with the factor that best represented that particular dimension. These questions had high content validity and explained 73.93% of the total variance.

Among the nine extracted factors, the first factor was titled post treatment aesthetic and social satisfaction. This covered the patient's satisfaction with the appearance of their treatment and whether this had a positive impact on their social interaction. Factor two covered the patient's knowledge of the implant and bridge treatment modalities. The third factor, the pre-treatment self-esteem factor, described the impact their missing tooth had on how the patient perceived themselves, their appearance and their interaction within social situations. Factor 4 was the procedural factor, which described the impact the different aspects of the specific dental procedures had on the patient's treatment choice. The fifth factor, the oral health belief factor described how important the patient believed oral health is, its importance in maintaining nutrition and its impact on general health. Factor 6 was pre-treatment functioning, which described the masticatory functioning of the patient prior to the replacement of their missing tooth. Functional satisfaction was the seventh factor, which referred to the patient's perceived improvement in masticatory functioning after the completion of their dental treatment. Factor 8 covered the patient's knowledge of the denture treatment option. The ninth and final factor, the post treatment economic satisfaction factor, described whether or not the patient believed that they received value for the cost of their dental treatment. SPSS was used to determine the validity and reliability of the questionnaire. A Cronbach α level of .86 was obtained indicating that the overall reliability level of the questionnaire was relatively high. The 9 extracted factors were also found to be reliable with levels ranging from .67 to .95.

These questions had high content validity and explained 73.93% of the total variance. This questionnaire was developed to assess communication in the dental encounter. More specifically, the researchers aimed to utilize the questionnaire to determine if dentists were engaging in SDM with their patients. The researchers also aimed to determine if those patients who experienced SDM as identified in the questionnaire had a higher knowledge of treatment alternatives and a higher sense of treatment satisfaction. The questionnaire showed good level of discriminant validity that it can sensitively differentiate the difference between the SDM group and comparison group in post treatment aesthetic and social satisfaction. That is, the SDM group had a significantly higher sense of post treatment aesthetic and social satisfaction than the comparison group. The SDM questionnaire can also differentiate the SMD group and comparison group in regards to the knowledge of other treatment modalities, with the SDM group having a higher level of knowledge than the comparison group. This result is consistent with other studies that indicate that effective SDM can be measured by examining the patient's overall knowledge of treatment options (19).

The results indicated that only 26.6% of participants were exposed to SDM. In regards to knowledge, no significant difference was seen between the two groups with respect to denture knowledge. This may be because the denture treatment modality is more widely known amongst the general population. Consequently, SDM is not required to provide sufficient knowledge of this treatment modality.

No difference was seen on other levels of satisfaction. While several studies have highlighted the link between SDM and increased satisfaction, other studies suggest otherwise (19). It has been suggested that when clinicians display uncertainty and do not specifically recommend a treatment option for the patient, satisfaction can be decreased (19). This is because the provision of treatment options and the uncertainty as to which treatment option to select can overwhelm and confuse patients (19). The use of satisfaction as the most appropriate outcome measure of an effective decision making process has subsequently been questioned (20).

Limitations

This study was limited to patients from a private dental practice and a university dental clinic in Australia. In order to better understand the dental encounter and the use of SDM within dental practice, a large sample size from a broad range of dental practices should be utilized and in addition to this, this study only examined the decision making process involved in a single tooth replacement. Exploring the decision making process of other clinical situations may further aid in understanding the decision making process in the dental encounter. Finally, this study focused on a single treatment decision. In order to gain better insight into the use of SDM within clinical dentistry, examination of the complete dental encounter from the initial consultation to completion of treatment, to long- term post treatment maintenance, may be required.

Conclusion

This study was the first to explore the use of SDM in clinical dental practice in regards to single tooth replacement. A questionnaire was developed and a nine factor structure was derived using the present sample. This suggests that a nine factor solution can be used to assess the decision making process in the dental encounter. In regards to examining the prevalence of SDM and its ability to improve patient's knowledge and satisfaction, further research is required using a large sample size from an increased number of dental practices. This study highlights the importance of SDM in dental practice and provides direction for further research into SDM in clinical dentistry.

References

[1] Frosch DL, Kaplan RM. Shared decision making in clinical medicine: past research and future directions. Am J Prev Med 1999;17(4):85-94.

[2] Butalid L, Verhaak PFM, Boeije HR, Bensing JM. Patients' views on changes in doctor-patient communication between 1982 and 2001: A mixed-methods study. BMC Fam Pract 2012;13:80.

[3] Benbassat J, Pilpel D, Tidhar M. Patients' preferences for participation in clinical decision making: a review of published surveys. Behav Med 1998;24(2):81-8.

[4] Matthias MS, Salyers MP, Frankel RM. Re-thinking shared decision-making: Context matters. Patient Educ Couns 2013, in press.

[5] Charles C, Gafni A, Whelan T. Shared decision-making in the medical encounter: what does it mean? (or it takes at least two to tango). Soc Sci Med 1997;44(5): 681-92.

[6] Joosten EAG, DeFuentes-Merillas L, de Weert GH, Sensky T, van der Staak CPF, de Jong CAJ. Systematic review of the effects of shared decision-making on patient satisfaction, treatment adherence and health status. Psychother Psychosom 2008;77(4):219-26.

[7] Elwyn G, Frosch D, Thomson R, Joseph-Williams N, Lloyd A, Kinnersley P, et al. Shared decision making: a model for clinical practice. J Gen Intern Med 2012;27(10):1361-7.

[8] Epstein RM, Street RLJr. Shared mind: communication, decision making, and autonomy in serious illness. Ann Fam Med 2011;9(5):454-61.

[9] Elwyn G, Miron-Shatz T. Deliberation before determination: the definition and evaluation of good decision making. Health Expect 2010;13(2):139-47.

[10] Montgomery AA, Harding J, Fahey T. Shared decision making in hypertension: the impact of patient preferences on treatment choice. Fam Pract 2001;18(3):309-13.

[11] Towle A, Godolphin W. Framework for teaching and learning informed shared decision making. BMJ 1999;319(7212):766-71.

[12] Savage R, Armstrong D. Effect of a general practitioner's consulting style on patients' satisfaction: a controlled study. BMJ 1990;301(6758):968-70.

[13] Sbaraini A, Carter SM, Evans RW, Blinkhorn A. Experiences of dental care: What do patients value? BMC Health Serv Res 2012;12:177.

[14] Newsome PR, Wright GH. A review of patient satisfaction: 2. Dental patient satisfaction: An appraisal of recent literature. Br Dent J 1999;186(4 Spec No): 166-70.

[15] Crow R, Gage H, Hampson S, Hart J, Kimber A, Storey L et al. The measurement of satisfaction with healthcare: implications for practice from a systematic review of the literature. Health Technol Assess 2002;6(32):1-244.

[16] Al-Quran FA, Al-Ghalayini RF, Al-Zu'bi BN. Single-tooth replacement: factors affecting different prosthetic treatment modalities. BMC Oral Health 2011;11:34.

[17] Hebel K, Gajjar R, Hofstede T. Single-tooth replacement: bridge vs. implant-supported restoration. J Can Dent Assoc 2000;66(8):435-8.

[18] MackF, Samietz SA, Mundt T, Proff P, Gedrange T, Kocher T, et al. Prevalence of single-tooth gaps in a population-based study and the potential for dental implants--data from the Study of Health in Pomerania (SHIP-0). J Craniomaxillofac Surg 2006;34(Suppl 2):82-5.

[19] Politi MC, Clark MA, Ombao H, DizonD, Elwyn G. Communicating uncertainty can lead to less decision satisfaction: a necessary cost of involving patients in shared decision making? Health Expect 2011;14(1):84-91.

[20] Sepucha K, Ozanne E, Silvia K, Partridge A, Mulley AG Jr. An approach to measuring the quality of breast cancer decisions. Patient Educ Couns 2007;65(2):261-9.

In: Health Promotion
Editors: J. Sun, N. Buys, J. Merrick
ISBN: 978-1-62257-870-2

Chapter VII

Association of shared decision-making to knowledge and treatment satisfaction in dental patients

***Jessica Peters, BA, BOralH*[1], *Jing Sun, PhD**[*2] *and Florian Mack, PhD*[1]**
[1]School of Oral Health and Dental Science, Griffith University, Centre for Medicine and Oral Health, Southport, Australia
[2]School of Public Health and Griffith Health Institute. Griffith University, Logan Campus, Meadowbrook, Australia

Abstract

Shared decision making (SDM) is an approach in which the clinician and patient go through all stages of the decision making process together. The use of SDM has been thoroughly explored in clinical medicine, however little research has examined SDM in dentistry. In this chapter we examine the use of SDM in patients who have received treatment for missing

* *Correspondence:* Jing Sun, PhD, School of Public Health, Griffith University and Griffith Health Institute, Griffith University, Gold Coast Campus, Parkland, Q4222 Australia. E-mail: j.sun@griffith.edu.au.

teeth. Method: A cross sectional study design was used to assess patients from a university dental clinic and a private dental practice. Patients were required to complete the SDM questionnaire. Results: Of the 144 participants, only 29.9% were exposed to SDM. The results of multiple linear regression suggested that the provision of SDM in the dental encounter, led to an increase in patient's knowledge of treatment alternatives and post treatment aesthetic/social satisfaction. However, the provision of SDM in the dental encounter did not lead to an increase in denture knowledge, post treatment functional satisfaction or post treatment economic satisfaction. Multiple linear regression also identified pre-treatment self esteem, oral health beliefs and attitudes and pre-treatment masticatory functioning as factors that mediate the relationship between SDM and the outcome variables. Conclusion: Decision-making in dentistry and the outcomes of dental treatment is a multifocal complex process. While this study demonstrates the importance of SDM in achieving favourable clinical outcomes, further research is required examining the interaction of patient factors with SDM. In order to further understand decision making in dentistry, further research should focus on examining the use of SDM in other facets of dentistry.

Introduction

Research has highlighted shared decision making (SDM) as a method to facilitate a strong clinician patient relationship (1,2). SDM is an approach in which the clinician and patient go through all phases of the decision making process together (1). When SDM is employed, information is provided about the health problem, the possible treatment options and consequences of the treatments are discussed, and together the clinician and patient consider how these fit with the patient's preferred outcomes (1). After all the options are considered, a decision is made based on mutual agreement (3).

The concept of SDM has been thoroughly explored in the medical literature with many benefits reported (2,4-12). Such benefits include improvements in; treatment adherence, patient knowledge, quality of life, satisfaction, general health and wellbeing. It is however evident that little research has examined SDM in the dental encounter (13). With many benefits reported in clinical medicine, it is proposed that dental patients would benefit greatly if SDM was implemented in the dental encounter. This study subsequently seeks to examine SDM in the dental encounter. More specifically, this study seeks to examine the use of SDM in patients who have received treatment for missing teeth and determine if SDM leads to increased knowledge and satisfaction. This study will provide evidence of the benefits obtained when SDM is employed in dentistry, specifically in patients seeking treatment for missing teeth. It is hoped that this study will demonstrate that similar benefits can be obtained when SDM is used in the dental setting as reported in the medical setting. This study will demonstrate that involving patients in the decision making process is critical in achieving successful clinical outcomes, with particular emphasis on increased dental knowledge and treatment satisfaction. This study is particularly important, as the use of SDM in dentistry has not yet been fully explored.

While this study seeks to demonstrate the importance of SDM in the dental encounter, it is recognized that multiple factors are at play. Mediating factors are expected to influence the relationship between SDM and dental knowledge and SDM and treatment satisfaction. These factors include: procedural factors, pre-treatment masticatory functioning, pre-treatment self-esteem and oral health beliefs/attitudes. These factors will be included in the current study. The aim of this study is to examine SDM in patients who have received dental treatment for missing teeth and to determine if SDM leads to increased dental knowledge and treatment satisfaction. This study also aims to identify factors that mediate the relationship between SDM and dental knowledge and SDM and treatment satisfaction. Specifically, the following objectives of the study will be examined: 1) To determine participants level of knowledge of dental treatment options via the implementation of the SDM questionnaire, 2) To determine participants level of post treatment satisfaction via the implementation of the SDM questionnaire, 3) To compare the SDM group and the comparison group on levels of knowledge of dental treatment options and post treatment satisfaction using linear regression and 4) To explore the mediating effects of procedural factors, oral health beliefs/attitudes, pre-treatment masticatory functioning, and pre-treatment self-esteem on the relationship between SDM and dental knowledge and SDM and satisfaction using linear regression.

The hypotheses of the study

- Patients who have experienced SDM have a higher level of knowledge of dental treatment options.
- Patients who have experienced SDM do not have a higher level of knowledge of dental treatment options.

- Patients who have experienced SDM have a greater sense of post treatment satisfaction.
- Patients who have experienced SDM do not have a greater sense of post treatment satisfaction.
- Procedural factors, oral health beliefs/attitudes, pre-treatment masticatory functioning, and pre-treatment self-esteem mediate the relationship between SDM and dental knowledge and SDM and treatment satisfaction.
- Procedural factors, oral health beliefs/attitudes, pre-treatment masticatory functioning, and pre-treatment self-esteem do not mediate the relationship between SDM and dental knowledge and SDM and treatment satisfaction.

Our study

A cross sectional study design was used to collect data from patients who either visited the Griffith University dental clinic or a private dental practice. Data was collected from December 2012 to May 2013. Patients who had received treatment for a tooth gap were invited to attend the study. A tooth gap is a gap resulting from a missing tooth that is bordered by one or more natural teeth on either side (14). Participants may have multiple missing teeth, however the presence of a tooth gap with either a single or double span is required. Two inclusion criteria were used. Participants must have received treatment for missing teeth and the treatment must have been completed. Participants were selected from the Griffith University dental clinic in Queensland and a private dental practice in Tasmania. Patients were identified via computer records. Informed consent has been obtained from both facilities. There were 144 dental patients invited to attend the study and all of them agreed to participate in the study with 100% response rate. Ethical approval has been obtained through Griffith University Ethics Committee.

Measures

A questionnaire has been developed to assess SDM in patients who have received treatment for missing teeth. A pilot study has been completed and necessary adjustments were made. The questionnaire includes 107 items.

Items are scored on either a 2 point scale (1, yes; 0, no) or on a 6 point scale (5, strongly agree; 4, agree; 3, some what agree; 2, some what disagree; 1, disagree; 0, strongly disagree). When asked about treatment alternatives, patients must rank their level of knowledge from 1 to 7. The reliability and validity of the SDM questionnaire has been established. A Cronbach α level of .86 was obtained indicating that the overall reliability of the questionnaire is high. The SDM questionnaire demonstrates high content validity (explaining 73.93% of the total variance) and discriminant validity (ability to distinguish the SDM group from the comparison group).

Outcome variables

Knowledge

The participant's knowledge of treatment alternatives was assessed using eight questions (question 64- 72). Three questions are present for each of the three treatment modalities: removable partial denture (acrylic or chrome cobalt denture), fixed dental prosthesis (bridge) and implant supported crown. Patients are required to rank their level of knowledge from 1 to 7. For example; did you know what an implant looked like before the completion of your treatment?

Treatment satisfaction

Treatment satisfaction is assessed on four levels; functional, aesthetic, social and economic satisfaction. Three items (90-92) assess functional satisfaction, which measure the patient's satisfaction with their post treatment masticatory functioning. For example: after the replacement of my missing tooth I can now eat crunchy fruit. Item 94-96 assess aesthetic satisfaction. This includes: after the replacement of my missing tooth I am happier with how my mouth looks. Social satisfaction is measured using items 96-99. For example: after the replacement of my missing tooth I now enjoy meeting new people. Economic satisfaction is measured using item 100 and 101. For example: I believe that I received value for the cost of my dental treatment.

Mediating variables

The questionnaire also examines procedural factors, oral health beliefs/attitudes, pre-treatment masticatory functioning and the patient's pre-treatment self-esteem. These factors may mediate the relationship between the independent and outcome variables.

Confounding factors

Demographic factors, which may confound the relationship between SDM and knowledge and SDM and satisfaction, will also be collated. This includes; age, gender, income, place of residence, level of education, family and general health status. Whether the patient's treatment was covered by private health insurance or government assistance will also be collated.

Procedure of data collection

Patients were approached in both the private and public dental clinics. They were provided with an information sheet outlining the purpose of the study and the study procedure. If patients agreed to participate they were provided with the questionnaire. Data was entered into SPSS.

Statistical analysis

SPSS version 22.0 was used to analyse the data. Factor analysis, Chi-square and multiple linear regression analysis were used to analyse the data.

Factor analysis, reliability and validity of the SDM questionnaire

Statistical analysis was conducted on unweighted data. A principle component analysis was conducted to investigate the subscales structure within the questionnaire. Varimax rotation was considered appropriate for the current study, which uses an orthogonal rotation method that minimizes the number of variables that have high loadings on each factor. Exploratory factor analysis was used to extract the factor structure of the questionnaire. Pearsons correlation bivariate analysis was completed to ensure each factor was not highly correlated and represented an independent concept. Reliability was also assessed from analyses of internal consistency using Cronbach α. A normality check was completed, and non-parametric tests applied to any factor that was not normally distributed.

Chi-square bivariate analysis

Chi-square bivariate analysis was completed to examine the differences between the SDM group and comparison group on demographic factors. Demographic factors that were included in the chi-square analysis included: age, gender, place of residency, level of education, income, general health, family status, and whether or not the patient received private health or government assistance for their dental treatment. If a significant difference was found the confounding factors were included in the multivariate analysis.

Multiple linear regressions

Multiple linear regressions were run to test the relationship between SDM and the dependent variables dental knowledge and treatment satisfaction. Three models were run for each linear regression in order to test the three research hypotheses.

H_1: Patients who have experienced SDM have a higher level of knowledge of dental treatment options.

To test hypothesis one, the multiple linear regression model was used to examine the relationship between the independent variable SDM and the dependent variable knowledge of dental treatment options. Confounding factors identified from the chi-square analysis were controlled in the model.

H_2: Patients who have experienced SDM have a greater sense of post treatment satisfaction.

To test hypothesis two, the multiple linear regression model was used to examine the relationship between the independent variable SDM and the dependent variable treatment satisfaction. Confounding factors identified from the chi-square analysis were controlled in the model.

H_3: Procedural factors, oral health beliefs/attitudes, pre-treatment masticatory functioning, and pre-treatment self-esteem mediate the relationship between SDM and dental knowledge and SDM and treatment satisfaction.

To test hypothesis three, the mediating factors were imputed into a separate block to see if they influence the relationship between the independent and dependent variables. Confounding factors identified from the chi-square analysis were controlled in the model. The level of significance to test research hypotheses is $p<0.05$.

Findings

The demographic characteristics of the sample are depicted in table 1 below. One hundred and forty four participants completed the survey with 100%

response rate. Of these participants, 50.0% were aged between 45-64 years, while 44.4% were aged 65 years and above and only 5.6 % aged less than 44 years. Among the respondents, 82 (56.9%) were female. Education levels indicated that 42.4 % had tertiary education, 16.0 % had diploma/training and further education, 40.3 % had secondary education and only 1.4 % had primary education level. When looking at place of residence, 107 (74.8%) were from metropolitan/city area, 30 (21.0%) from a semi rural area and 6 (4.2%) from a rural area. In terms of family status, 107 (74.8 %) were living in a relationship/partnership and 36 (25.0%) were single. When look at average household income, 30.4% of participants reported earning $37,000 or less, 34.8% reported $37,001- $80,000, 29.0% reported $80,001- $180,000, and 5.8% reported $180,001 and over per year.

Table 1. Demographic characteristics of the sample

Categorical Variable	N (%)
Age	
>44 years	8 (5.6%)
45- 64 years	72 (50.0%)
65 years and over	64 (44.4%)
Gender	
Male	62 (43.1%)
Female	82 (56.9%)
Education level	
Primary education	2 (1.4%)
Secondary education	58 (40.3%)
Diploma/tafe	23 (16.0%)
Tertiary education	61 (42.4%)
Place of residency	
Metropolitan/city area	107 (74.8%)
Semi rural area	30 (21.0%)
Rural area	6 (4.2%)
Family status	
Living in a relationship/partnership	107 (74.8%)
Single	36 (25.0%)
Household income	
<$37,000	42 (30.4%)
$37,001- $80,000	48 (34.8%)
$80,001- $180,000	40 (29.0%)
>$180,001	8 (5.8%)

Dental characteristics of the sample

As seen in table 2 below, 105 (72.9%) participants received private health insurance for their dental treatment whereas 27 (18.8%) received government assistance for their dental treatment. Thirty (20.8%) participants from the total sample reported that they had previously been treated for gum disease. In regards to the number of missing teeth, 52 (36.1%) had only 1 missing tooth, 35 (24.5%) had 2-3 missing teeth and 56 (39.2%) had more than 3 missing teeth.

Table 2. Dental characteristics of participants

Variable	N (%)
Private health insurance	
Yes	105 (72.9%)
No	39 (27.1%)
Government assistance	
Yes	27 (18.8%)
No	117 (81.3%)
Gum Disease	
Yes	30 (20.8%)
No	114 (79.2%)
Number of missing teeth before treatment	
Only one missing tooth	52 (36.1%)
2-3 missing teeth	35 (24.5%)
> 3 missing teeth	56 (39.2%)
Location of missing tooth	
Front	89 (61.8%)
Middle	48 (33.3%)
Back	36 (25.0%)
Can your missing tooth be seen when you smile	
Yes	98 (68.1%)
No	46 (31.9%)
Cause of tooth Loss	
Trauma/accident	40 (27.8%)
Tooth decay	50 (34.7%)
Gum disease	10 (6.9%)
Root resorption	7 (4.9%)
Failed dental treatment	25 (17.4%)
Tooth never formed	9 (6.3%)
Tooth was impacted	9 (6.3%)
Cracked tooth	27 (18.8%)
Unsure	9 (6.3%)
How long the tooth was missing before seeking treatment	
< 3 months	88 (61.1%)
3-6 months	11 (7.6%)
6 months -1 year	4 (2.8%)
1-3 years	13 (9.0%)
> 3 years	30 (20.8%)
Final treatment choice	
CrCo RPD	39 (27.1%)
Acrylic RPD	14 (9.7%)
Implant supported crown	45 (31.3%)
FPD	48 (33.3%)

When looking at the location of the missing teeth, 89 (61.8%) participants indicated that their missing tooth/teeth was located at the front of their mouth, with 98 (68.1%) participants indicating that their missing tooth/teeth could be seen when they smiled. The most commonly reported cause of tooth loss was; decay (34.7%), trauma (27.8%), cracked tooth (18.8%) and failed dental treatment (17.4%). Nine (6.3%) participants were unsure of the cause of their missing tooth/teeth. When looking at how long the patient waited before seeking treatment, 88 (61.1%) sought treatment immediately, 15 (10.4%) sought treatment within one year, 13 (9.0%) sought treatment within 1-3 years and, 30 (20.8%) waited more than 3 years for treatment. Finally, when looking at the final treatment choice, 48 (33.3%) participants received a fixed dental prosthesis, 39 (27.1%) participants received a chrome cobalt denture, 14 (9.7%) participants received an acrylic denture, and 45 (31.3%) participants received an implant-retained crown.

Grouping of participants

Whether or not alternative treatment options were discussed with patients by their dentist was examined. It was found that only 43 (29.9%) participants were presented with all three treatment options and could subsequently be assigned to the SDM group. Twenty-five (17.7%) participants were presented with two treatment options, 73 (51.8%) participants were presented with one treatment option and two (1.4%) participants were not presented with any treatment options. These participants were assigned to the comparison group.

Dependent and mediating variables

The mean and standard deviation of the dependent and mediating variables are presented in table 3 below. As all variables are normally distributed (see table 4), presentation of the mean and standard deviation is most appropriate.

Factor analysis

Factor analysis needed to be completed on the SDM questionnaire before the hypothesis could be tested and the relationship between SDM and dental knowledge and SDM and treatment satisfaction could be determined. Factor analysis was completed on the items in the SDM questionnaire in order to classify the variables into more meaningful categories.

Table 3. Mean and standard deviation of the dependent and mediating variables

Dependent Variables	Mean (SD)
Knowledge of treatment alternatives	19.40 (13.15)
Denture knowledge	15.00 (6.50)
Post- treatment aesthetic/social satisfaction	24.05 (8.81)
Post-treatment functional satisfaction	12.37 (3.57)
Post-treatment economic satisfaction	7.17 (2.39)
Mediating Variables	**Mean (SD)**
Procedural factors	6.90 (6.21)
Pre-treatment masticatory functioning	11.15 (5.67)
Pre-treatment self esteem	13.79 (9.59)
Oral health beliefs/attitudes	23.05 (2.47)

Table 4. Skewness and kurtosis of dependent and mediating variables

Variable	Skewness (standard error)	Kurtosis (standard error)
Knowledge of treatment alternatives	0.791 (0.206)	-0.638 (0.408)
Denture knowledge	-0.682 (0.205)	-0.985 (0.407)
Post- treatment aesthetic/social satisfaction	-0.554 (0.205)	-0.869 (0.407)
Post-treatment functional satisfaction	-1.813 (0.206)	0.076 (0.410)
Post-treatment economic satisfaction	-0.568 (0.206)	-0.627 (0.408)
Procedural factors	1.134 (0.206)	1.569 (0.408)
Pre-treatment masticatory functioning	-0.195 (0.207)	-1.002 (0.411)
Pre-treatment self esteem	0.634 (0.207)	-0.652 (0.411)
Oral health beliefs/attitudes	-1.203 (0.206)	0.745 (0.408)

The Exploratory Factor Analysis derived a nine component solution from the factor analysis (see appendix 1). Pre-treatment self-esteem was the first factor, which included 7 items 80, 85, 86, 87, 88, 89 and 90. For example; before my treatment I did not like meeting new people, and I did not feel good about myself. Factor 2 was knowledge of the two other treatment modalities; implant retained crown and fixed dental prosthesis. This was assessed using items 67, 68, 69, 70, 71, 72 and 73. Factor 3 [Items 94, 95, 96, 97, 98, 99] indicated the respondent's level of post treatment aesthetic and social satisfaction. For example: after the replacement of my missing tooth I feel more confident. Factor 4 represented the degree to which procedural factors impacted on the patient's treatment choice. This was measured using items 74, 75, 76, 77, 78 and 79. The fifth factor comprised the oral health beliefs/attitudes of the patient. This was measured using items 102, 103, 104, 106, and 107 such as: I believe that good teeth are important for general health. Factor 6 included items 81, 82, 83, and 84, which measured pre-treatment masticatory functioning. Factor 7 measured patient's satisfaction with post treatment masticatory functioning [91,92,93]. The eighth factor expressed the patient's level of denture knowledge, which was assessed using items 64, 65, and 66. The ninth and final factor was post treatment economic satisfaction. This was measured using item 100 and 101.

Pearson's correlation bivariate analysis

Pearson's correlation bivariate analysis was completed to ensure each factor was not highly correlated (correlation < .85) and therefore represented an independent concept (see table 5). The variance explained by the nine factors were 11.28%, 11.15%, 11.10%, 8.03%, 7.51%, 7.08%, 6.40%, 6.04%, and 3.96% respectively. The total variance explained by the 9 factors was 72.54%.

Reliability of the SDM questionnaire

The overall reliability level of the questionnaire was relatively high with a Cronbachα level of 0.860. Tablc 6 below indicates that the subscales based on the 9 extracted factors were generally found to be reliable with levels ranging from 0.798 to 0.954.

Chi-square test

For the current study, a Chi-square test was used to describe the demographic characteristics of the SDM group and the comparison group and to compare the differences between them. The results are presented in table 7 below.

Table 5. Inter-correlation between the nine factors obtained from factor analysis

	Post treatment physical and social satisfaction	Post treatment functional satisfaction	Post treatment economic satisfaction	Denture knowledge	Knowledge of other treatment modalities	Pre-treatment self esteem	Pre-treatment functioning	Procedural factors
Post treatment physical and social satisfaction	.258**	0.161						
Post treatment functional satisfaction	0.117	0.035	0.114					
Post treatment economic satisfaction	.197*	0.036	-0.007	.292**				
Denture knowledge	.463**	0.072	0.128	-0.015	-0.128			
Knowledge of other treatment modalities	0.019	.196*	-0.103	-0.024	0.021	.272**		
Pre-treatment self esteem	0.011	-0.065	-0.117	0.05	-0.044	.205*	.191*	
Pre-treatment functioning	.379**	0.118	.209*	.219**	0.132	0.117	-0.067	-0.072

** Correlation is significant at the 0.01 level (2-tailed).

Table 6. Reliability correlations, Cronbach α

Questionnaire	Reliability correlations, Cronbach α (9 factors)
Total score	0.860
Pre-treatment self esteem	0.913
Knowledge of other treatment modalities	0.918
Post treatment aesthetic/social satisfaction	0.916
Procedural factors	0.806
Oral health beliefs	0.798
Pre-treatment functioning	0.850
Post treatment functional satisfaction	0.954
Denture knowledge	0.914
Post treatment economic satisfaction	0.695

Table 7. Chi-square analysis to identify confounding factors

Variable	Group Comparison group N(%)	SDM group (%)	χ^2	P value
age			3.262	0.353
<25	1 (100%)	0 (0%)		
25-44	3 (42.9%)	4 (57.1%)		
45- 64	50 (69.4%)	22 (30.6%)		
>64	47 (46.5%)	17 (39.5%)		
Gender			4.070	**0.044****
Male	38 (61.3%)	24 (38.7%)		
Female	63 (76.8%)	19 (23.2%)		
Place of residency			1.081	0.583
Metropolitan	78 (72.9%%)	29 (27.1%)		
Semi rural	19 (63.3%)	11 (36.7%)		
Rural	4 (66.7%)	2 (33.3%)		
Level of education			0.403	0.940
Primary	1 (50.0%)	1 (50.0%)		
Secondary	41 (70.7%)	17 (29.3%)		
Diploma/tafe	16 (69.6%)	7 (30.4%)		
Teriary	43 (70.5%)	18 (29.5%)		
Family status			0.120	0.729
Single	26 (72.2%)	10 (27.8%)		
Living in a relationship/partnership	74 (69.2%)	33 (30.8%)		

Variable	Group Comparison group N(%)	SDM group (%)	χ^2	P value
Household income			3.589	0.464
0-18,200	3 (75.0%)	1 (25.0%)		
18,201-37,000	30 (78.9%)	8 (21.1%)		
37,001-80,000	34 (70.8%)	14 (29.2%)		
80,001- 180,000	24 (60.0%)	16 (40.0%)		
>180,000	5 (62.5%)	337.5%)		
General health			4.756	0.191
Poor	2 (100%)	0 (0%)		
Good	47 (73.4%)	17 (26.6%)		
Very good	32 (60.4%)	21 (39.6%)		
Excellent	20 (80.0%)	5 (20.0%)		
Private health insurance				
Yes	73 (69.5%)	32 (30.5%)	0.070	0.791
No	28 (71.8%)	11 (28.2%)		
Government assistance			0.246	0.620
Yes	20 (74.1%)	7 (25.9%)		
No	81 (69.2%)	36 (30.8%)		

**P< 0.05.

The demographic factor of gender was significance (*p*= 0.044). This indicates that there is not equal distribution between the comparison group and the SDM group in regards to this variable. Gender is therefore a confounding factor that has the potential to influence the relationship between the independent and dependent variables. Gender will subsequently be included in the multiple linear regression. A non-significant result (*p*>0.05) was found for the variables of age, place of residency, education, family status, household income, general health, private health insurance and government assistance. This indicates that these variables are represented equally in both the SDM group and the comparison group.

Multiple linear regression

From factors analysis, the dependent variable knowledge was broken down into two factors; denture knowledge and knowledge of the other treatment alternatives. The dependent variable treatment satisfaction was broken down into; post treatment aesthetic/social satisfaction, post treatment functional satisfaction and post treatment economic satisfaction. Subsequently, linear regression was run for each of the five dependent variables produced from factor analysis. Three models were run for each of the five dependent variables.

The relationship between SDM and knowledge of treatment alternatives

As demonstrated in table 8 below, SDM had a positive relationship with knowledge of treatment alternatives. That is, the provision of SDM in the dental encounter, lead to an increase in knowledge of treatment alternatives. SDM had a regression coefficient value of 6.501 (95% CI: 1.763, 11.238) demonstrating a significant positive influence of knowledge of treatment alternatives (*p*=0.008).

Table 8. The relationship between SDM and knowledge of treatment alternatives

Predictor Variable	Regression coefficient (95% CI)	P value
SDM	6.501 (1.763, 11.238)	**0.008****

Table 9 below, displays the influence SDM had on knowledge of treatment alternatives, when the mediating factors and confounding factor gender were also considered. Even when including the mediating and confounding factors, SDM still had a significant positive influence on knowledge of treatment alternatives (*p*=0.017). This level of significance was however slightly lower, when these additional factors were included. When looking at the influence the mediating factors had on knowledge of treatment alternative, it appears that pre-treatment self-esteem (*p*= 0.050) and oral health beliefs/attitudes (*p*= 0.024) were significant mediators of the relationship between SDM and knowledge of treatment alternatives. Pre-treatment self-esteem had a regression coefficient value of 0.243 (95% CI: -0.003, 0.489) demonstrating a significant positive mediating relationship. That is, as the pre-treatment self-esteem of the patient increased, knowledge of treatment alternatives also increased. A significant mediating effect was also seen for oral health beliefs/attitudes with a regression coefficient of 1.161 (95% CI: 0.159, 2.164) demonstrating a significant positive mediating influence on knowledge of treatment alternatives. That is, as the oral health belief/attitudes of the patient increased, knowledge of treatment alternatives also increased. The mediating factors; pre-treatment functioning and procedural factors, as well as the confounding factor gender did not appear to be strong mediators in the relationship between SDM and knowledge of treatment alternatives as indicated by non significant *p* values.

Table 9. The influence of SDM, mediating factors and confounding factors on knowledge of treatment alternatives

Predictor variable	Regression coefficient (95% CI)	P value
Independent variable		
SDM	5.903 (1.057, 10.749)	**0.017****
Mediating factors		
Pre treatment self esteem	0.243 (-0.003, 0.489)	**0.050****
Procedural factors	-0.102 (-0.465, 0.262)	0.581
Oral health beliefs/attitudes	1.161 (0.159, 2.164)	**0.024****
Pre-treatment functioning	-0.171 (-0.647, 0.306)	0.480
Confounding factors		
Gender	-3.029 (-8.064, 2.005)	0.236

**P< 0.05.
Correlation coefficient (R): 0.343.
Adjusted R squared: 0.075.
ANOVA F value: 2.792**.

The ANOVA F ratio for the model was 2.792. This was statistically significant with a *p* value <0.05. This indicates that the prediction of the X/Y relationship was significant. The adjusted R-squared value was 0.075. This suggests that 7.5% of the variance in knowledge of treatment alternatives is explained by SDM, the mediating factors and the confounding factor gender.

The relationship between SDM and denture knowledge

As demonstrated in table 10 below, SDM did not appear to be a strong predictor of denture knowledge (p=0.644).

Table 10. The relationship between SDM and denture knowledge

Predictor Variable	Regression coefficient (95% CI)	P value
SDM	0.564 (-1.847, 2.976)	0.644

As demonstrated in table 11 below, even when taking into account the influence of mediating and confounding factors, SDM still was not found to be a strong predictor of denture knowledge (p= 0.664). That is, the provision of SDM in the dental encounter, did not lead to an increase in denture knowledge. When looking at the mediating factors, pre treatment self esteem (p=0.579), procedural factors (p=0.490), and pre-treatment functioning (p=0.961) did not significantly mediate the relationship between SDM and denture knowledge. The mediating factor oral health beliefs/attitudes was however significant (p= 0.020) with a regression coefficient of 0.612 (95% CI: 0.100, 1.125). As the regression coefficient was positive it was suggested that as the oral health beliefs/attitudes of the patient increased, the denture knowledge of the patient also increased. Finally, gender (p= 0.737) was not found to significantly predict denture knowledge.

Table 11.The influence of SDM, mediating factors and confounding factors on denture knowledge

Predictor variable	Regression coefficient (95% CI)	P value
Independent variable		
SDM	0.544(-1.931, 3.020)	0.664
Mediating factors		
Pre treatment self esteem	0.033 (-0.090, 0.162)	0.579
Procedural factors	0.065 (-0.121, 0.251)	0.490
Oral health beliefs/attitudes	0.612 (0.100, 1.125)	**0.020****
Pre-treatment functioning	-0.012 (-0.211, 0.201)	0.961
Confounding factors		
Gender	0.438 (-2.135, 3.010)	0.737

**P< 0.05.

Correlation coefficient (R): 0.252.

Adjusted R squared: 0.019.

ANOVA F value: 0.213.

The ANOVA F ratio for the model was 0.213. This was not statistically significant. The adjusted R-squared value was 0.019. This suggests that only 1.9% of the variance in denture knowledge is explained by SDM, the mediating factors and the confounding factor gender.

The relationship between SDM and post-treatment aesthetic/social satisfaction

As demonstrated in table 12 below, SDM had a positive relationship with post-treatment aesthetic/social satisfaction. SDM had a regression coefficient value of 3.873 (95% CI: 0.752, 6.993) demonstrating a significant positive influence on post-treatment aesthetic/social satisfaction (*p*=0.015). That is, the provision of SDM in the dental encounter, lead to an increase in post treatment aesthetic/social satisfaction.

Table 12. The relationship between SDM and post treatment aesthetic/social satisfaction

Predictor Variable	Regression coefficient (95% CI)	P value
SDM	3.873 (0.752, 6.993)	**0.015****

Table 13 below, displays the influence SDM had on post-treatment aesthetic/social satisfaction, when the mediating factors and confounding factor gender were also considered. As shown in table 13, even when examining the influence of the mediating and confounding factors, SDM still had a significant positive influence on post-treatment aesthetic/social satisfaction (*p*=0.023). This level of significance was however slightly lower, when these additional factors were also included. When looking at the influence the mediating factors had on the relationship between SDM and post-treatment aesthetic/social satisfaction, it appears that pre-treatment self-esteem (*p*<0.001) and oral health beliefs/attitudes (*p*<0.001) demonstrated a significant effect. Pre-treatment self-esteem had a regression coefficient value of -0.413 (95% CI: -0.546, -0.275) demonstrating a significant negative relationship. That is, when the pre-treatment self-esteem of the patient decreased, the post-treatment aesthetic/social satisfaction increased. A significant predictive effect was also seen for oral health beliefs/attitudes with a regression coefficient of 1.258 (95% CI: 0.703, 1.814) demonstrating a significant positive influence on post-treatment aesthetic/social satisfaction. That is, as the oral health belief/attitudes of the patient increased, post-treatment aesthetic/social satisfaction also increased. The mediating factors pre-treatment functioning and procedural factors, as well as the confounding factor gender did not appear to influence the relationship between SDM and post treatment aesthetic/social satisfaction as indicated by non significant *p* values.

The ANOVA F ratio for the model was 12.227. This was statistically significant with a *p* value <0.001. This indicates that the prediction of the X/Y relationship was significant. The adjusted R-squared value was 0.336. This suggests that 33.6% of the variance in post treatment aesthetic/social satisfaction is explained by SDM, the mediating factors and the confounding factor gender.

Table 13. The influence of SDM, mediating factors and confounding factors on post-treatment aesthetic/social satisfaction

Predictor variable	Regression coefficient (95% CI)	P value
Independent variable		
SDM	3.123 (0.437, 5.809)	**0.023****
Mediating factors		
Pre treatment self esteem	-0.413 (-0.546, -0.275)	**<0.001*****
Procedural factors	-0.154 (-0.355, 0.047)	0.132
Oral health beliefs/attitudes	1.258 (0.703, 1.814)	**<0.001*****
Pre-treatment functioning	0.107 (-0.156, 0.371)	0.423
Confounding factors		
Gender	-2. 363 (-5.154, 0.427)	0.096

**P< 0.05 ***P< 0.001.

Correlation coefficient (R): 0.605.

Adjusted R squared: 0.336.

ANOVA F value: 12.227***.

The relationship between SDM and post-treatment functional satisfaction

As demonstrated in table 14 SDM did not appear to be a strong predictor of post-treatment functional satisfaction (p=0.134).

Table 14. The relationship between SDM and post treatment functional satisfaction

Predictor Variable	Regression coefficient (95% CI)	P value
SDM	0.945 (-0.293, 2.183)	0.134

As demonstrated in table 15 even when taking into account the influence of mediating and confounding factors, SDM still was not found to be a strong predictor of post treatment functional satisfaction (p= 0.216). That is, the provision of SDM in the dental encounter, did not lead to an increase in post treatment functional satisfaction. The mediating factor pre-treatment functioning had a regression coefficient value of -0.160 (95% CI: -0.283, -0.037) demonstrating a significant negative relationship (p= 0.011). That is, pre-treatment functioning was shown to mediate the relationship between SDM and post treatment functional satisfaction. As the regression coefficient was negative it is suggested that as the pre-treatment functioning of the patient decreased, the post treatment functional satisfaction increased. The other mediating factors: pre treatment self esteem (p=0.870), procedural factors (p=0.087) and oral health beliefs/attitudes (p=0.141) did not influence the relationship between SDM and post-treatment functional satisfaction. Finally, gender (p=0.751) did not significantly predict post treatment functional satisfaction.

Table 15. The influence of SDM, mediating factors and confounding factors on post-treatment functional satisfaction

Predictor variable	Regression coefficient (95% CI)	P value
Independent variable		
SDM	0.791 (-0.467, 2.049)	0.216
Mediating factors		
Pre treatment self esteem	-0.005 (-0.069, 0.058)	0.870
Procedural factors	-0.082 (-0.176, 0.012)	0.087
Oral health beliefs/attitudes	0.195 (-0.065, 0.455)	0.141
Pre-treatment functioning	-0.160 (-0.283, -0.037)	**0.011****
Confounding factors		
Gender	-0.210 (-1.517, 1.098)	0.751

**P< 0.05.
Correlation coefficient (R): 0.310.
Adjusted R squared: 0.053.
ANOVA F value: 2.248**.

The ANOVA F ratio for the model was 2.248. This was statistically significant with a p value <0.05. This indicates that the prediction of the X/Y relationship was significant. The adjusted R-squared value was 0.053. This suggests that 5.3% of the variance in post treatment functional satisfaction is explained by SDM, the mediating factors and the confounding factor gender.

The relationship between SDM and post-treatment economic satisfaction

As demonstrated in table 16 below, SDM did not appear to be a strong predictor of post treatment economic satisfaction (p=0.681).

Table 16. The relationship between SDM and post treatment economic satisfaction

Predictor Variable	Regression coefficient (95% CI)	P value
SDM	-0.182 (-1.057, 0.692)	0.681

As demonstrated in table 17 below, even when taking into account the influence of mediating and confounding factors, SDM still was not found to be a strong predictor of post treatment economic satisfaction (p= 0.724). That is, the provision of SDM in the dental encounter, did not lead to an increase in post treatment economic satisfaction. When looking at the mediating factors, pre-treatment self esteem (p=0.043) did have a significant mediating effect (95% CI: -0.090, 0.001) on the relationship between SDM and post treatment economic satisfaction. This is represented by a negative regression coefficient, which indicates that as the pre-treatment self esteem of the patient decreased, their post treatment economic satisfaction increased. All of the other mediating factors, procedural factors (p=0.189), oral health beliefs/attitudes (p=0.111) and pre-treatment functioning (p=0.491) as well as gender (p= 0.795) did not significantly influence the relationship between SDM and post treatment economic satisfaction.

Table 17. The influence of SDM, mediating factors and confounding factors on post-treatment economic satisfaction

Predictor variable	Regression coefficient (95% CI)	P value
Independent variable		
SDM	-0.159 (-1.050, 0.731)	0.724
Mediating factors		
Pre treatment self esteem	-0.044 (-0.090, 0.001)	**0.043****
Procedural factors	-0.044 (-0.111, 0.022)	0.189
Oral health beliefs/attitudes	0.149 (-0.035, 0.333)	0.111
Pre-treatment functioning	0.036 (-0.052, 0.123)	0.419
Confounding factors		
Gender	-0.210 (-1.045, 0.802)	0.795

**P< 0.05.

Correlation coefficient (R): 0.268.

Adjusted R squared: 0.028.

ANOVA F value: 1.625**.

The ANOVA F ratio for the model was 1.625. This was statistically significant with a p value <0.05. This indicates that the prediction of the X/Y relationship was significant. The adjusted R-squared value was 0.028. This suggests that 2.8% of the variance in post treatment economic satisfaction is explained by SDM, the mediating factors and the confounding factor gender.

Discussion

Exploratory factor analysis in the current study showed a 9 factor solution, suggesting that 9 factor can be used to assess the patient's experience in the dental encounter specifically relating to the treatment of missing teeth. The Cronbach α level of 0.86 indicated that the overall reliability level of the questionnaire was high. The 9 extracted factors were also found to be reliable with levels ranging from 0.798 to 0.954. These questions had high content validity and explained 72.54% of the total variance. Subsequently it is concluded that the SDM questionnaire is a valid and reliable measure of SDM in patients who have received treatment for missing teeth.

SDM and knowledge

The results of linear regression suggested that the provision of SDM in the dental encounter was associated with increased knowledge of other treatment alternatives. This result is consistent with other studies that indicate that effective SDM can be measured by examining the patient's overall knowledge of treatment options (15). However, SDM was not associated with increased denture knowledge. This finding may be explained by the fact that the denture treatment modality is more widely known amongst the general population. It is possible that SDM is not required for this type of knowledge to be obtained.

The oral health beliefs and attitudes of a patient were a significant predictor for both knowledge of other treatment alternatives and denture knowledge. This is consistent with research that suggests that patients with strong oral health beliefs are more motivated to understand their oral health conditions and how their health status can be improved (16). Finally, self-esteem was a significant mediator in the relationship between SDM and knowledge of other treatment modalities. It was found that patients with low self-esteem prior to dental treatment had lower knowledge of treatment options following treatment. This is consistent with research that suggests that low self-esteem and psychological dysfunction can hinder an individual's ability to retain new information (17).

SDM and post treatment satisfaction

This study demonstrated that the provision of SDM in the dental encounter was associated with an increase in post treatment aesthetic/social satisfaction. This finding supports Swanson et al (18) who concluded that involving patients in treatment decisions and providing a thorough explanation, leads to increased satisfaction (18). However in the current study, SDM was not associated with increased post treatment economic or functional satisfaction.

When looking at the influence the mediating factors had on post treatment satisfaction, the pre treatment self esteem of the patient was found to be significantly related to post treatment aesthetic/social satisfaction and post treatment economic satisfaction. It was found that patients with low self esteem prior to dental treatment, reported higher levels of aesthetic/social satisfaction and economic satisfaction following treatment. The presence of missing teeth can negatively impact on a patients psychological and social functioning and may act as a barrier to personal and social success (19,20). Patients with greater psychosocial impairment attributed to unfavourable dentition, have greater clinical outcomes following prosthodontics rehabilitation and this is supported in the current study (21).

The oral health beliefs of the patient were found to be significantly related to post treatment aesthetic/social satisfaction. This suggests that the oral health beliefs of a patient can impact their treatment outcomes. The current study subsequently supports researchers who suggest that patients with strong oral health beliefs are more likely to appreciate the changes obtained following treatment and report greater levels of satisfaction (22).

Finally, the pre treatment functioning of a patient was found to be significantly related to post treatment functional satisfaction. The results of the linear regression suggested that patients with impaired masticatory functioning prior to treatment, reported greater post treatment functional satisfaction. The results of the current study are consistent with studies that suggest that patients with greater functional impairment prior to treatment will have greater clinical outcomes following prosthodontics rehabilitation (21).

Limitations

There are a number of limitations for this study. Selection bias may have been present in the current study, as it did not have blind selection. Random sampling would be a method to overcome selection bias. Allocation to the

SDM group and the comparison group was based upon participants recognising the use of SDM in the interaction with their dentist and reporting this in the questionnaire. Some measurement bias may have been present if patients failed to indicate that SDM had been used if in fact it had. Finally, analysis bias may have occurred when entering data into SPSS. However, cleaning the data would help overcome this bias. In order to reduce the occurrence of random error, increasing the sample size is required.

As data is only collected from two dental clinics, the generalizability of the results is limited. The researchers made every effort to improve this by selecting patients who had received different treatment options for their missing teeth and participants from a wide range of backgrounds. The fact that the study included both private and public dental patients does improve the generalizability of the results. However, in order to improve the generalizability of these results and to gain a better insight into the use of SDM in dentistry a large sample size from a broader range of dental practices should be utilized. In addition to this, this study only examines SDM in tooth replacement. Exploring SDM in other clinical situations may further aid in understanding the decision-making process in the dental encounter.

Conclusion

In conclusion it is evident that decision making in dentistry and the outcomes of dental treatment is a complex process and multiple factors are at play. While SDM is important in achieving favourable treatment outcomes, It is suggested that further research is required examining the interaction of patient factors with SDM. Perhaps the use of SDM in combination with encouraging patients to have strong oral health beliefs and attitudes and helping to improve patients self esteem would aid in achieving more successful clinical outcomes including patient's dental knowledge and patient satisfaction.

Appendix 1. Principle component analysis for nine-factor structure

	Pre treatment self esteem	Knowledge of other treatment modalities	Post treatment social/ aesthetic satisfaction	Procedural factors	Oral health beliefs	Pre-treatment functioning	Post treatment functional satisfaction	Denture knowledge	Post treatment economic satisfaction
Before my treatment I did not like meeting new people.	**.877**	-.073	.165	.168	-.012	.077	.008	.066	.089
Before my treatment I did not feel good about myself.	**.861**	-.069	.138	.097	.066	.165	.029	-.073	.098
Before my treatment I felt that people were staring at my missing tooth.	**.850**	-.042	.251	.100	-.054	.020	-.030	-.040	.052
Before my treatment I did not like speaking in public.	**.850**	-.098	.135	.136	-.034	.104	-.012	.100	.079
Before my treatment I lacked confidence.	**.820**	-.072	.142	.078	.007	.233	.000	-.145	.147
Before my treatment I was unhappy with how my mouth looked.	**.720**	-.093	.310	.029	.036	.153	-.021	.027	-.162
A major reason for the replacement of my missing tooth was my appearance.	**.434**	-.013	.225	-.122	.225	-.235	.159	.155	-.244

	Pre treatment self esteem	Knowledge of other treatment modalities	Post treatment social/ aesthetic satisfaction	Procedural factors	Oral health beliefs	Pre-treatment functioning	Post treatment functional satisfaction	Denture knowledge	Post treatment economic satisfaction
Did you know how an implant was inserted before your treatment?	-.046	**.878**	.105	-.059	.010	.085	-.003	.080	-.213
Did you know how to clean an implant before your treatment?	-.009	**.877**	.126	-.064	-.010	.105	-.042	.102	-.093
Did you know how a bridge was constructed before your treatment?	-.109	**.873**	.078	-.018	.101	-.104	.092	.067	.172
Did you know what an implant looked like before your treatment?	-.033	**.865**	.106	-.084	-.014	.114	.055	.043	-.221
Did you know how to clean a bridge before your treatment?	-.084	**.837**	.068	.027	.109	-.059	.076	.113	.159
Did you know what a bridge looked like before your treatment?	-.177	**.766**	.015	-.052	.138	-.152	.161	.134	.097
Damage to the surrounding teeth through drilling was a factor that influenced my final treatment choice.	.081	**.410**	-.105	.391	.103	.182	-.179	.058	.161
After the replacement of my missing tooth I feel more confident.	.192	.068	**.858**	.045	.167	.002	.123	-.073	.059

Appendix 1. (Continued)

	Pre treatment self esteem	Knowledge of other treatment modalities	Post treatment social/ aesthetic satisfaction	Procedural factors	Oral health beliefs	Pre-treatment functioning	Post treatment functional satisfaction	Denture knowledge	Post treatment economic satisfaction
After the replacement of my missing tooth I feel better about myself.	.174	.082	**.827**	.033	.088	.077	.137	.015	.189
After the replacement of my missing tooth I now enjoy meeting new people.	.285	.109	**.825**	-.002	.039	-.020	.066	.122	.092
After the replacement of my missing tooth I feel more comfortable smiling.	.181	.079	**.822**	-.132	.166	-.100	.064	.038	.063
After the replacement of my missing tooth I am happier with how my mouth looks.	.128	-.022	**.809**	-.115	.179	-.101	.160	-.058	-.076
After the replacement of my missing tooth I now enjoy speaking in public.	.329	.160	**.736**	-.009	.049	-.013	.054	.149	.071
I believe that missing or decayed teeth are a sign of poor health.	-.050	.244	**.413**	.068	.390	.134	-.110	-.061	.165

	Pre treatment self esteem	Knowledge of other treatment modalities	Post treatment social/ aesthetic satisfaction	Procedural factors	Oral health beliefs	Pre-treatment functioning	Post treatment functional satisfaction	Denture knowledge	Post treatment economic satisfaction
The amount of pain I associated with each procedure influenced my final treatment choice.	.147	-.107	-.042	**.870**	.024	.080	.057	-.065	.069
The amount of discomfort I associated with each procedure influenced my final treatment choice.	.038	-.130	-.008	**.812**	.047	.134	.019	.003	.050
I experience fear/anxiety towards dental treatment and this influenced my final treatment choice.	.110	-.164	-.011	**.797**	.045	.132	-.008	.025	-.037
Duration of the treatment was a factor that influenced my final treatment choice.	.095	.185	-.035	**.692**	-.240	.001	-.016	.000	.044
Cost of the treatment was a factor that influenced my final treatment choice.	-.111	-.053	-.082	**.567**	-.152	-.030	-.149	.100	-.178
The materials that are used in each procedure were a factor that influenced my final treatment choice.	.183	.070	.064	**.533**	.107	.045	-.055	.011	-.131
I believe that good teeth are important for my general health.	-.084	.053	.093	.006	**.865**	-.020	.148	.117	.016

Appendix 1. (Continued)

	Pre treatment self esteem	Knowledge of other treatment modalities	Post treatment social/ aesthetic satisfaction	Procedural factors	Oral health beliefs	Pre-treatment functioning	Post treatment functional satisfaction	Denture knowledge	Post treatment economic satisfaction
I believe that good teeth are important for eating and chewing.	.002	.060	.031	-.094	**.753**	.113	.083	.033	.078
I believe that someone with all their teeth looks better than someone with missing teeth.	.036	.025	.053	-.065	**.725**	-.086	.032	.157	.007
I believe good teeth are important for maintaining nutrition.	.016	.161	.208	.100	**.690**	.014	-.030	-.002	.003
I believe that good teeth are important for my appearance	.153	-.071	.345	-.017	**.642**	-.235	-.044	.132	.031
Before my treatment I found it difficult to eat crunchy fruit.	.167	-.040	.054	.105	-.046	**.886**	.120	.023	-.047
Before my treatment I found it difficult to eat crunchy vegetables.	.201	.022	.056	.124	-.050	**.879**	.067	-.033	.011
Before my treatment I found it difficult to eat cooked meat.	.212	-.016	-.032	.149	-.096	**.869**	.079	.032	.004

	Pre treatment self esteem	Knowledge of other treatment modalities	Post treatment social/aesthetic satisfaction	Proce dural factors	Oral health beliefs	Pre-treatment functioning	Post treatment functional satisfaction	Denture know ledge	Post treatment economic satisfaction
A major reason for the replacement of my missing tooth was my ability to eat and chew.	-.002	.085	-.180	.022	.109	**.528**	.128	-.050	-.175
After the replacement of my missing tooth I can now eat crunchy fruit.	.020	.056	.092	-.054	.042	.128	**.930**	-.009	.071
After the replacement of my missing tooth I can now eat crunchy vegetables.	.015	.086	.158	-.077	.046	.118	**.925**	.011	.088
After the replacement of my missing tooth I can now eat cooked meat.	-.021	.083	.193	-.029	.091	.136	**.874**	.084	.088
Did you know how to use a denture before your treatment?	-.013	.193	-.003	.050	.121	.004	.075	**.921**	.054
Did you know how to clean a denture before your treatment?	.026	.131	.009	.059	.093	.011	-.009	**.915**	.153
Did you know what a denture looked like before your treatment?	-.011	.146	.104	-.020	.161	-.047	.014	**.842**	-.116
I believe I paid too much reversed	.108	-.084	.120	-.105	.013	-.054	.121	.049	**.792**
I believe that I received value for the cost of my dental treatment.	.109	.054	.251	-.030	.168	-.152	.134	.048	**.733**

References

[1] Frosch DL, Kaplan RM. Shared decision making in clinical medicine: past research and future directions. Am J Prev Med 1999;17(4):285-94.

[2] Joosten EA, DeFuentes-Merillas L, de Weert GH, Sensky T, van der Staak CP, de Jong CA. Systematic review of the effects of shared decision-making on patient satisfaction, treatment adherence and health status. Psychother Psychosom 2008;77(4):219-26.

[3] Charles C, Gafni A, Whelan T. Shared decision-making in the medical encounter: what does it mean? (or it takes at least two to tango). Soc Sci Med 1997;44(5):681-92.

[4] Adams JR, Drake RE, Wolford GL. Shared decision-making preferences of people with severe mental illness. Psychiatr Serv 2007;58(9):1219-21.

[5] Clever SL, Ford DE, Rubenstein LV, Rost KM, Meredith LS, Sherbourne CD, et al. Primary care patients' involvement in decision-making is associated with improvement in depression. Med Care 2006;44(5):398-405.

[6] Deyo RA, Cherkin DC, Weinstein J, Howe J, Ciol M, Mulley AG, Jr. Involving patients in clinical decisions: impact of an interactive video program on use of back surgery. Med Care 2000;38(9):959-69.

[7] Gattellari M, Butow PN, Tattersall MH. Sharing decisions in cancer care. Soc Sci Med 2001;52(12):1865-78.

[8] Greenfield S, Kaplan S, Ware JE, Jr. Expanding patient involvement in care. Effects on patient outcomes. Ann Intern Med 1985;102(4):520-8.

[9] Hamann J, Cohen R, Leucht S, Busch R, Kissling W. Shared decision making and long-term outcome in schizophrenia treatment. J Clin Psychiatry 2007;68(7):992-7.

[10] Morgan MW, Deber RB, Llewellyn-Thomas HA, Gladstone P, Cusimano RJ, O'Rourke K, et al. Randomized, controlled trial of an interactive videodisc decision aid for patients with ischemic heart disease. J Gen Intern Med 2000;15(10):685-93.

[11] Ruland CM, White T, Stevens M, Fanciullo G, Khilani SM. Effects of a computerized system to support shared decision making in symptom management of cancer patients: preliminary results. J Am Med Inform Assoc 2003;10(6):573-9.

[12] van Roosmalen MS, Stalmeier PF, Verhoef LC, Hoekstra-Weebers JE, Oosterwijk JC, Hoogerbrugge N, et al. Impact of BRCA1/2 testing and disclosure of a positive test result on women affected and unaffected with breast or ovarian cancer. Am J Med Genet Part A 2004;124A(4):346-55.

[13] Johnson BR, Schwartz A, Goldberg J, Koerber A. A chairside aid for shared decision making in dentistry: a randomized controlled trial. J Dent Educ 2006;70(2):133-41.

[14] Mack F, Samietz SA, Mundt T, Proff P, Gedrange T, Kocher T, et al. Prevalence of single-tooth gaps in a population-based study and the potential for dental implants--data from the Study of Health in Pomerania (SHIP-0). J Craniomaxillofac Surg 2006;34(Suppl 2):82-5.

[15] Politi MC, Clark MA, Ombao H, Dizon D, Elwyn G. Communicating uncertainty can lead to less decision satisfaction: a necessary cost of involving patients in shared decision making? Health Expect 2011;14(1):84-91.

[16] Broadbent JM, Thomson WM, Poulton R. Oral health beliefs in adolescence and oral health in young adulthood. J Dent Res 2006;85(4):339-43.

[17] Whitesell NR, Mitchell CM, Spicer P. A longitudinal study of self-esteem, cultural identity, and academic success among American Indian adolescents. Cultur Divers Ethnic Minor Psychol 2009;15(1):38-50.

[18] Swanson KA, Bastani R, Rubenstein LV, Meredith LS, Ford DE. Effect of mental health care and shared decision making on patient satisfaction in a community sample of patients with depression. Med Care Res Rev 2007;64(4):416-30.

[19] Chen P, Yu S, Zhu G. The psychosocial impacts of implantation on the dental aesthetics of missing anterior teeth patients. Br Dent J 2012;213(11):E20.

[20] Kerosuo H, Hausen H, Laine T, Shaw WC. The influence of incisal malocclusion on the social attractiveness of young adults in Finland. Eur J Orthodont 1995;17(6):505-12.

[21] Ozhayat EB. Influence of self-esteem and negative affectivity on oral health-related quality of life in patients with partial tooth loss. Community Dent Oral Epidemiol 2012.

[22] Reifel NM, Rana H, Marcus M. Consumer Satisfaction. Adv Dent Res 1997;11(2):281-90.

In: Health Promotion
Editors: J. Sun, N. Buys, J. Merrick

ISBN: 978-1-62257-870-2

Chapter VIII

Impact of stress on depression and anxiety in dental students and professionals

Christine Farrelly, BOralH[1], Jing Sun, PhD*[*2] and Florian Mack, PhD[1]

[1]School of Oral Health and Dental Science, Griffith University, Centre for Medicine and Oral Health, Southport, Australia
[2]School of Public Health and Griffith Health Institute. Griffith University, Logan Campus, Meadowbrook, Australia

Abstract

Recent evidence has highlighted stress and poor mental health as risk factors for further physical and psychological illness. Dental students have frequently been shown to suffer higher prevalence of stress and psychological dysfunction, though few studies use relevant comparison groups when reporting these measures. In this chapter we aim to examine the difference in psychological dysfunction between dental students and students in other disciplines. Questionnaires were distributed to cohorts

---

* *Correspondence:* Jing Sun, PhD, and Griffith Health Institute andSchool of Public Health, Griffith University, Griffith University, Gold Coast Campus, Parklands, QLD, 4222 Australia. Email: j.sun@griffith.edu.au

of dental students, undergraduate students and dental professionals around Australia. The DASS-21 was used to assess all participants' depression and anxiety and a modified version of the Dental Environmental Stress Questionnaire (DES) called the Student Environmental Stress (SES) Scale was used to assess students stress only. Demographic details for all participants were also collected. Dental students were significantly more stressed than dentists, and there were also significant difference between anxiety and depression between the three groups. Dental students only had significantly higher scores on one aspect of the extracted SES components. Linear regression showed a consistent significant relationship between student stress and all aspects of psychological dysfunction. The results of this study indicate that dental students do suffer higher psychological stress then dentists in the workforce. It also demonstrates the stress levels of dental students had higher level stress than undergraduate students in other discipline in academic study. The relationship between high student stress and psychological dysfunction enforces the importance of employing stress reduction program in the context of Australian universities and in particular dental students' academic program.

Introduction

Mental health and its impact on an individual's physical and psychological morbidity is important public health issue (1). Researchers have suggested a causal link between mental strains and an increased risk of morbidity (2), so early intervention is paramount. It has been well documented in the literature that dental students suffer from high levels of stress throughout their education (3). Associations between specific dental stressors and enhanced anxiety and depressive symptomology have also been demonstrated (4,5). A recent review by Alzahem (6) indicated that the major sources of stress faced by dental students were living accommodation factors, personal factors, educational environment factors, academic factors and clinical factors. It can be seen in the review that many of the major sources of stress for dental students can actually be relevant to most university students. Issues relating to these factors may be pertinent to most undergraduates and mental health issues faced by undergraduate students have also often been demonstrated in the literature (7,8). In past research though, psychological issues faced by dental students often lacked a representative comparison group (9).

It is a common conception among the general population that Dentists have one of the highest rates of suicide of any profession and a number of articles have been written about this apparent phenomenon with conflicting reports (10,11). Irrefutable though, are the high levels of stress faced by Dentists and this has been well documented for many years (12,13). How does the mental health of dental professionals compare to their university years though? A review of the literature found that studies comparing these cohorts were rare (14). A comparison of Dentists mental health with a cohort of dental students would help to determine if any theme of psychological dysfunction pertinent in University dissipates after graduation or if those in the dental industry are destined to be perpetually under strain.

The methodology of the proposed study allows for investigation into the correlation between mental health and personal factors and offers important contribution to mental health research. The use of novel self-report measures will allow the relationship between student stress and mental health to be explored. To the knowledge of the researchers, the proposed measures have yet to be employed in dental students or dental professionals and the correlations between these measures will help in understanding the relationship between stress and mental health in these cohorts.

This study aims to provide a meaningful reflection of the mental health of dental students by recruiting a sample of undergraduate students as a realistic baseline. It is postulated that the true levels of stress may in fact be altered when a general student population is included. Overall, the study will provide information regarding the mental health issues affecting dental students and dental professionals in Australia. If a relationship between student stress and psychological dysfunction is found, it will provide evidence that stress is detrimental to a student's health. Practically, it will provide a focus for policy-makers within the University environment to develop intervention and prevention programs tailored to the needs of specific students. This will allow for mental health issues faced by future students to be prevented before they lead to physical and psychological morbidity.

The present study will ask the following research questions; Are dental students more stressed, depressed and anxious than dental professionals and other undergraduate students? And are perceived student stressors and coping mechanisms associated with mental health?

To answer the research questions, specific aims have been developed for the study. The overall study aims are to compare the difference between dental students and professionals in psychological problems and to examine the association between stress, coping strategies and mental health in students and dental professionals in Australia. To answer the research questions and in accordance with the aims of the study the following hypotheses have been developed:

H_1: There are differences in the stress, anxiety and depression levels among dental students, undergraduate university students and dental professionals.

H_2: Dental students have higher perceived student stress than other undergraduate students.

H_3: Higher perceived student stress is associated with higher levels of psychological dysfunction.

Our study

Cross sectional study design was used for the study. Participants were sampled from a population of students attending University's in Queensland, primarily around the South East region. A quota sampling method was used, defining university students and dental students as the subgroups of interest and convenience sampling of each subgroup took place. Students were approached while at university and participation was completely voluntary. Any undergraduate students who were selected will be invited to attend this study. Students who were at post graduate level, on exchange program, were under the age of 17 due to consent issues, and external students due to difficulty in contact for this study were not invited to attend the study.

Dental Professional sample were approached from the wider community and Universities around Australia in attempts to achieve a representative sample population for comparability and generalizability. The sampling strategy was similar to the strategy employed to recruit the students, with convenience sampling of the accessible subpopulation. Surveys were handed out in person to Dentists in the southeast Queensland region and were collected immediately or returned to the researchers via mail. Questionnaires also were mailed out to Dentists working in other parts of Australia where prior permission has first been sought. All Dentists and Dental Specialists were invited to fill out the questionnaire, though Dental Assistants and Dental Hygienists who were not included in the study.

Informed consent was obtained from student sample and dental professionals, and ethics approval was obtained from Griffith University Ethics Committee (DOH/04/13/HREC).

Measures

DASS-21 (15)

The major variables of interest in the current study include levels of stress, anxiety and depression as measured by the DASS-21. The DASS-21 is a shortened version of a self-report questionnaire (DASS-42) developed by Australian Psychologists (15). The measure consists of seven questions specific for each measure and asks for symptoms experienced over the past week. Responses are scored on a four point Likert Scale from '0 = did not apply to me at all' to '3 = applied to me very much, or most of the time' (See Appendix 1). Depression, anxiety and stress scores can be described as normal, mild, moderate, severe or extremely severe depending on participants' total score for each item. The DASS-21 is a reliable and valid self-report measure that has been successfully employed previously in a variety of clinical and non-clinical samples (16, 17). Studies have found that the shortened version has advantages over the 42-item version, including a cleaner factor structure and smaller inter-factor correlations (18). Psychometric properties of the shortened scale have been verified in numerous studies and the questionnaire has been determined to have discriminate and construct validity and excellent internal consistency (18-21). The scale has shown to effectively differentiate between diagnostic groups and show correlations with other existing measures for similar constructs (18, 20).

Modified Dental Environmental Stress Questionnaire – Student Environmental Stress Questionnaire

In order to also gain a greater insight into the perceived sources of stress specifically faced by students, a modified version of the Dental Environmental Stress (DES) Scale will be used (22). The original scale developed by Garbee et al. (22) has been used successfully and consistently to measure perceived sources of stress in Dental Students and other professional students numerous times, both in its original format and modified versions (4, 9, 23, 24). For the proposed study, some items on the DES were modified in a similar way to those utilized by Murphy, Grey and colleagues (9). In order to pertain information regarding to stressors that may be faced by all undergraduate students, the questions were revised so that they applied to both groups. The survey was first reduced to thirty items after omitting questions relating specifically to patient and clinical responsibilities. Secondly, the questions that pertained specifically to Dentistry were altered to reflect a general university environment. For example, a question on the original DES that asked, "lack of confidence to be a successful dentist" became "lack of confidence to be a successful graduate (See appendix 2 for omitted and altered questions). It was ensured that the essential purpose of the question remained intact and the altered questions were reviewed and approved by the researchers to ensure their face validity as predictors of undergraduate stress. The 30 remaining questions asked students to indicate the level of stress associated with each item on a Likert Scale of '1= not stressful' to '4= very stressful' and fifth option indicating the question was irrelevant. The questionnaire was termed the Students Environmental Stress (SES) Scale.

Coping and demographics

The participants surveyed will also be asked about the coping strategies they use in times of stress, both positive and negative. Additional demographic and socio-economic variables were also collected in the survey questionnaire. This included general data on age, income and living arrangements. Specific demographics relating to students and dental professionals were also asked.

Statistical analysis

The statistical package for social sciences (SPSS) will be used for data processing and data analyses. Dimension reduction of the DASS-21 will completed based previous models of the instrument and factor analysis of the modified DES will be conducted to condense the data and allow for ease of interpretation. Validity will be determined for each measure by determining Cronbachs alpha for each sub-population in the study. A chi-square test will be undertaken to present the demographic data and to determine any differences between the groups in these factors. Comprehensive analysis of the data will depend on the specific hypotheses under investigation.

Hypothesis 1: Dental students have higher stress, anxiety and depression levels than other undergraduate university students and dental professionals.

To test the first hypothesis, a multivariate analysis of variance (MANOVA) or equivalent non-parametric test will be carried out to determine any differences in the dependent variable, psychological disturbance among the grouping variable which is participants profession (Dentist, dental student or undergraduate student).

Hypothesis 2: Dental students have higher perceived stress than other undergraduate students.

An Independent samples t-test will be carried out to determine differences in student stress between dental students and other undergraduate students.

Hypothesis 3: Higher perceived student stress is associated with higher psychological distress.

A multiple linear regression model will be used to determining the relationship between the independent variable, students perceived stress from the SES with the dependent variable, student scores on the DASS-21. The influence of demographic variables and other factors will also be determined by including them as confounding variables in the analysis.

The level of significance to test the hypotheses for the current study was set $p>0.05$.

Our findings

Statistical assumption check

The analytical assumptions for the current study depended on the hypothesis being tested and statistical test being carried out. Firstly the data was checked to identify and outliers or invalid values. It was found that one participant's data (ID 30) contained an outlier in the DASS-21 measure; this was checked and corrected. Assumptions were met for the dimension reduction for both measures (DASS-21 and SES Scale) and Factor Analyses were carried out. The DASS-21 data was reduced in accordance with previous psychometric analyses (18, 20) and the components and their internal reliability is shown below in Appendix 1. Factor analysis for the SES scale yielded four components, with a Bartlett's test of sphericity was significant ($p<0.001$) and the measure of sampling adequacy was 0.786, which is sufficient.

Assumptions for Pearson's correlation were met as data was entered as a Likert scale and are linearly related to one another. Data was also checked for extreme outliers. A Pearson's Correlation was carried out on the factors for each measure to confirm that they were not highly correlated. Each measure was below 0.80 confirming independence of components for both the DASS-21 and the SES Scale. The three groups included in the analysis are dental professionals, dental students and undergraduate students and each are sufficiently independent of each other. The dependent variables included are depression, anxiety and stress and were normally distributed as shown by skewness and kurtosis between -3 and +3. Levene's test of variance was completed and it was determined that homogeneity of variance in the groups could be assumed for the measure of stress only. The measures of anxiety and depression had a p-value below 0.05 and therefore the assumption for a MANOVA could not be met for these measures. Due to this assumption of variance not being met, a non-parametric test must be used, Kruskal-Wallis in this case. Kruskal-Wallis test uses median instead of means and determines rank differences between the groups as an extension of a Mann-Whitley test.

The two groups being tested in the t-test are dental students and undergraduate students and the dependant variable is perceived stress on a student stress scale. For the t-test, the dependant variable had to be normally distributed. This was checked by determining that the skewness and kurtosis for the four factors discovered by means of factor analysis were all within the range of -3 to 3. As they were, a t-test is a suitable analysis. Variance within the groups was determined by Levene'e test for Equality of Variances, and t-values and significance were determined accordingly.

For the final statistical model, multiple linear regression analysis, the relationship between student stress and psychological dysfunction is approximately linear as demonstrated by a scatter plot (data not shown). It is an assumption while running a multiple linear regression model that the DV is normally distributed. In the case of the current study the DV's are stress, anxiety or depression as measured by the DASS-21. These are normally distributed as shown in Appendix 4. The IV's are continuous in regards to student stress levels, so they may be entered directly into the regression model. Categorical confounding factors and coping mechanisms need to be transformed to be included in the regression.

Descriptive analysis results

After cleaning the data the final sample contained valid data from 153 participants. In regards to the explanatory variable, data was collected from 78 Dental Students, 54 undergraduate students and 21 Dental professionals.

Table 1. Overall demographics for the sample

Demographic Variable	N (%)
Gender	
Male	70 (45.8)
Female	83 (54.2)
Living arrangement	
Living alone	6 (3.6)
Share house	70 (45.8)
Living with Family	56 (36.6)
Living with Partner	21 (13.7)
Income	
1-5999	61 (39.9)
6000-19999	57 (37.3)
20000-59999	17 (11.1)
60000-99999	4 (2.6)
100000 +	14 (9.2)
Smoking	
no	134 (90.3)
former	6 (4.1)
yes	8 (5.4)
Alcohol	
no	42 (28)
yes	108 (72)

Table 2. Student demographics

Demographic Variable	N (%)
Year of study	
1st	34 (26.6)
2nd	28 (21.9)
3rd	15 (11.7)
4th	25 (19.5)
5th	26 (20.3)
Study load	
Full time	124 (96.9)
Part time	4 (3.1)
GPA	
0-3.9	3 (2.7)
4-4.9	11 (9.7)
5-5.9	36 (31.9)
6-7	63 (55.8)
Prior study	
Secondary	58 (45.3)
Diploma/TAFE	7 (5.5)
Incomplete bachelors	43 (33.6)
Bachelors	15 (11.7)
Postgraduate	5 (3.9)

Table 3. Dental professional demographics

Dentists demographic characteristics	N (%)
How long employed	
1-5	4 (20)
6-10	2 (10)
over 10	14 (70)
Completion of degree	
Australia	14 (73.7)
Overseas	5 (26.3)
Role in dental field	
Principal dentist	2 (10.5)
General dentist	10 (52.6)
Specialist	7 (36.8)

Table 4. Cohort Demographics

Sample Variables	Dentist N (%)	Dental student N (%)	Student N (%)	Total N (%)
Gender				
Male	12 (17.1)	28 (40)	30 (42.9)	70 (45.8)
Female	9 (10.8)	50 (60.2)	24 (28.9)	83 (54.2)
Living arrangement				
Living alone	1 (16.7)	3 (50)	2 (33.3)	6 (3.6)
Share house	0	50 (71.4)	20 (28.6)	70 (45.8)
Living with Family	11 (19.6)	16 (28.6)	29 (51.8)	56 (36.6)
Living with Partner	9 (42.9)	9 (42.9)	3 (14.3)	21 (13.7)
Income				
1-5999	0	37 (60.7)	24 (39.3)	61 (39.9)
6000-19999	0	32 (56.1)	25 (43.9)	57 (37.3)
20000-59999	3 (17.6)	9 (52.9)	5 (29.4)	17 (11.1)
60000-99999	4 (100)	0	0	4 (2.6)
100000 +	14 (100)	0	0	14 (9.2)
Smoking				
no	17 (12.7)	68 (50.7)	49 (36.6)	134 (90.3)
former	2 (33.3)	2 (33.3)	2 (33.3)	6 (4.1)
yes	1 (12.5)	6 (75)	1 (12.5)	8 (5.4)
Alcohol				
no	5 (11.9)	18 (42.9)	19 (45.2)	42 (28)
yes	15 (13.9)	59 (54.6)	34 (31.5)	108 (72)

The median age of the entire sample was 22 years (17-68). Within in the sample, 86 (55.1%) were females and 70 (44.9%) were males. The majority of the sample were non-smokers (90.5%) and 72% said that they drank alcohol.

The demographic and descriptive statistics for categorical data for the entire sample are shown below in Tables 1 to 3.

There are three groups in the current study. In addition to the entire samples descriptive statistics shown above, the demographics for each group are presented below in Table 4.

Table 5. Psychological dysfunction as measured by DASS-21

	Cohort		
	Dentist	**Student**	**Dental Student**
Depression	3.9 (4.2)	10.52 (9.41)	9.95 (9.45)
Anxiety	3.2 (3.87)	7.67 (7.07)	9.5 (8.66)
Stress	9.62 (6.47)	13.37 (9.8)	16.75 (9.98)

Table 6. Perceived Student stress scores as measured by the SES Scale

	Student group	
	Undergraduate student	**Dental student**
Home and relationship	5.96 (4.99)	6.02 (5.8)
School and faculty	12.86 (4.06)	18.5 (5.43)
Finance and future	12.07 (3.63)	13.4 (4.22)
Time and workload	18.75 (4.22)	18.61 (5.42)

Table 7. Continuous variables among the cohorts- Age and leisure activities

	Dentist M (SD)	**Undergraduate Student M (SD)**	**Dental student M (SD)**
Age [a b]	43.53 (13.7)	20.57 (4.8)	23.05 (3.6)
Gym/Working out	2.3 (1.8)	2.6 (2.7)	2.6 (1.8)
Team/Individual sport [a b]	0.52 (1.03)	1.33 (2.05)	2.7 (1.8)
Catching up with friends	1.9 (1.16)	1.33 (2.06)	2.7 (1.85)
Leisure activities: Beach/shopping [a b]	1.67 (1.56)	1.87 (1.68)	1.1 (1.2)
Movie/TV	0.4 (0.58)	1.07 (1.6)	1.12 (1.46)
Music	0.95 (1.6)	1.3 (2.27)	1.26 (2.34)
Studying [a]	0.95 (1.6)	1.37 (2.27)	1.2 (2.3)
Sleeping	7.1 (1.3)	7.3 (1.45)	7.1 (1.2

[a] $p<0.05$ between three groups

[b] $p<0.05$ between student and dental student.

In order to describe the outcome variables, the average scores on the DASS-21 for each group are shown below in Table 5. In regards to students and their stressors, the average values are shown in Table 6.

Potential confounding factors are determined by means of a Chi-square test for categorical variables or by ANOVA or t-test for continuous variables. Descriptive statistics for continuous and potentially confounding factors are shown below in Table 7. The Chi-square analysis for determining confounding factors among categorical variables is shown in Table 8.

An ANOVA showed that there was a significant difference between the groups for team or individual sports, leisure activities, studying and age. (Data not shown). In relation to hypothesis three, which focuses specifically on students, a t-test revealed that there were significant difference between student groups in leisure activities, team/individual sport and age (data not shown). Also in regards to hypothesis three, a separate Chi-square test needed to be carried out comparing categorical demographics among the student groups only. This test revealed that there were significant differences among these groups in the factors of 'Gender', 'Prior study', 'GPA', 'Year of study' and 'Living arrangement'. Results are also shown in Table 8.

Associations between potential confounding variables and both outcome variables

Factor analysis was firstly completed to reduce the data so hypothesis testing could be carried out. The results of factor analysis and their reliability are shown in Appendix 1 and 2 for the two measures used. Pearson's Correlation was also carried out to determine that none of the variables used were too highly correlated; the results of this analysis are shown in Appendix 3. After these analyses were carried out it was then possible to explore the associations between potential confounding variables and outcome and explanatory variables.

Within the current study, there is the possibility that certain demographic factors may be under or overexpressed in certain cohorts. If this is the case, these variables are referred to as confounding factors, as they may confound the relationship between the variables and elicit unwanted effects. These factors should therefore be included in relevant statistical analyses. The confounding factors within the current study depend on the variable type and the specific hypothesis.

The categorical demographic data among the three groups that may have an influence on the first hypothesis are shown below in table 8. The Chi-square analysis revealed that there were disproportionate amounts of males and females among the three groups (x^2=6.241, p=0.044). It was also found that more students lived in share houses when compared to Dentists (x^2=43.433, p<0.001) and that Dentists earned significantly more money (x^2=132.595, p<0.001). Smoking and alcohol use were similar throughout the three groups. A one-way ANOVA was used to determine if there were significant differences in the continuous variables between the three groups (see table 7 above). It was found that the Dental professional group was significantly older than both the dental student and undergraduate student group (p<0.05). There were significant differences between the three groups in the amount of times per week they engaged in team or individual sports and leisure activities such as shopping (p<0.05). Also, not surprisingly there was a significant difference between Dental Professionals and both student groups in how often they studied (p<0.05).

The second hypothesis explores the bivariate relationship between undergraduate students and dental students in regards to their stress levels. The potential categorical confounding factors are again revealed by Chi-square test and shown in Table 9 below. It was found that males and females where not distributed evenly between the groups (x^2=5.006, p=0.032). Significantly more dental students were found to be in later years of study (x^2=66.026, p<0.001) and they also had higher GPA's (x^2=44.924, p<0.001). Prior study was also disproportionate between the groups (x^2=29.037, p<0.001) as was living arrangement (x^2=15.977, p=0.001), though income and study load were similarly distributed. Continuous variables that were also significantly different have been revealed via a t-test and are shown above in Table 7. The amount of times per week the students engage in team sports and leisure activities like beach or shopping is significantly different (p<0.05) and dental students are also significantly older (p<0.05).

The effect of confounding variables can only be specifically revealed when running certain analyses. In the case of the statistical analyses used to address the first two hypotheses, confounding factors can be identified via a Chi-square test, though any effect they elicit cannot be statistically tested as they can't be inserted into the model. However, in the case of the linear regression model in the current study, which explores the relationship between student stress and psychological dysfunction, the influence of confounding factors may actually be measured. Confounding factors identified through Chi-square analysis (Table 9) or t-test (Table 7) may be entered directly into the model and it may be seen if these factors influence the relationship between the IV and the DV. This is a great advantage of a multiple linear regression model. The confounding factors identified between undergraduate students and dental students are mentioned above; gender, year of study, GPA, prior study and living arrangement were the categorical variables that have to be transformed before entering them into the regression. The continuous confounding factors of age, team sports and leisure activities can be directly entered in the model.

The linear regression models, which explore associations between potential confounding factors and both outcome and explanatory variables, are shown below in Table 13 to 15. The first linear regression (Table 13) explores the association between student stress and depression. Higher stress was significantly related to depression with a regression coefficient of 0.130 (95% CI= 0.073-0.186) ($p<0.001$). It was found the confounding factors of age (regression coefficient -0.274, 95% CI= -0.554-0.006) and living with family (regression coefficient -2.491, 95% CI= -4.446—0.536) had a significant protective effect on the relationship between student stress and depression levels ($p<0.05$). All other confounding factors were not significant. Table 14 demonstrates that student stress predicts anxiety with a regression coefficient of 0.138 (95% CI= 0.088-0.188) with a significance of $p<0.001$. It can be seen that confounding factors do not have any significant influence on the relationship. Finally Table 15 explores the predictive relationship between student stress and psychological stress. It shows that student stress significantly predicts psychological stress with a regression coefficient of 0.137 (95% CI= 0.088-0.186) ($p<0.001$). In regards to confounding factors, it can be seen that student stress is more predictive of psychological stress for females, with a regression coefficient of 2.914 (95%CI=1.296-4.533) ($p<0.05$). However, engaging in leisure activities has a significant negative relationship ($p<0.05$), indicating a protective influence on the student stress-psychological stress relationship (Regression coefficient -0.559, 95%CI= -1.066- -0.051). No other confounding factors reached significance.

Confounding factors results

A Chi Square test was completed to determine if any categorical demographic variables were confounding factors. The results of the Chi-square are shown in Table 8 for the entire sample and in Table 9 for determining confounding factors pertinent to the linear regression models.

Table 8. Chi-square test to determine confounding factors between the three groups

Sample Variables	Dentist N (%)	Dental student N (%)	Student N (%)	Total	x^2	p-value
Gender					**6.24**	**.044**
Male	12 (17.1)	28 (40)	30 (42.9)	70 (45.8)		
Female	9 (10.8)	50 (60.2)	24 (28.9)	83 (54.2)		
Living arrangement					**43.43**	**p<0.001**
Living alone	1 (16.7)	3 (50)	2 (33.3)	6 (3.6)		
Share house	0	50 (71.4)	20 (28.6)	70 (45.8)		
Living with Family	11 (19.6)	16 (28.6)	29 (51.8)	56 (36.6)		
Living with Partner	9 (42.9)	9 (42.9)	3 (14.3)	21 (13.7)		
Income					**132.59**	**p<0.001**
1-5999	0	37 (60.7)	24 (39.3)	61 (39.9)		
6000-19999	0	32 (56.1)	25 (43.9)	57 (37.3)		
20000-59999	3 (17.6)	9 (52.9)	5 (29.4)	17 (11.1)		
60000-99999	4 (100)	0	0	4 (2.6)		
100000 +	14 (100)	0	0	14 (9.2)		
Smoking					**4.33**	0.363
no	17 (12.7)	68 (50.7)	49 (36.6)	134 (90.3)		
former	2 (33.3)	2 (33.3)	2 (33.3)	6 (4.1)		
yes	1 (12.5)	6 (75)	1 (12.5)	8 (5.4)		
Alcohol					**2.53**	0.283
no	5 (11.9)	18 (42.9)	19 (45.2)	42 (28)		
yes	15 (13.9)	59 (54.6)	34 (31.5)	108 (72)		

Table 9. Chi-square test to determine confounding factors between the student groups

Student variables	Dental student N (%)	Student N (%)	Total	x^2	p-value
Gender				**5.006**	**0.032**
male	28 (48.3)	30 (51.7)	58		
female	50 (67.6)	24 (32.4)	74		
Year of study				**66.026**	**p<0.001**
1st	2 (5.9)	32 (94.1)	34		
2nd	17 (60.7)	11 (39.3)	28		
3rd	11 (73.3)	4 (26.7)	15		
4th	21 (84)	4 (16)	25		
5th	26 (100)	0	26		
Study load				**.380**	0.538
full time	74 (59.7)	50 (40.3)	124		
part time	3 (75)	1 (25)	4		
GPA				**44.924**	**p<0.001**
0-3.9	0	3 (100)	3		
4-4.9	0	11 (100)	11		
5-5.9	19 (52.8)	19 (52.8)	36		
6-7	56 (88.9)	7 (11.1)	63		
Prior study				**29.037**	**<0.001**
Secondary	24 (41.4)	34 (58.6)	58		
Diploma/TAFE	1 (14.3)	6 (85.7)	7		
Incomplete bachelors	36 (83.7)	7 (16.3)	43		
Bachelors	13 (86.7)	2 (13.3)	15		
Postgraduate	3 (60)	2 (40)	5		

Student variables	Dental student N (%)	Student N (%)	Total	x^2	p-value
Income				**0.423**	0.809
1-5999	37 (60.7)	24 (39.3)	61		
6000-19999	32 (56.1)	25 (43.9)	57		
20000-59999	9 (64.3)	5 (35.7)	14		
60000-99999	0	0			
Living arrangement				**15.977**	**0.001**
Living alone	3 (40)	2 (40)	5		
Share house	50 (71.4)	20 (28.6)	70		
Living with Family	16 (35.6)	29 (64.4)	45		
Living with Partner	9 (75)	3 (25)	12		

Table 10. Differences in student stress between undergraduate students and dental students

Variable	Student group		*t*	p-value
	Dental Student Mean (SD)	Undergraduate Student Mean (SD)		
Home and relationship	6.03 (5.8)	6.15 (5.035)	0.130	0.897
School and faculty	18.5 (5.4)	12.8 (4.11)	-6.337	<0.001***
Finance and future	13.4 (4.2)	12 (3.6)	-1.971	0.051
Time and workload	18.6 (5.4)	18.4 (4.1)	-0.241	0.810

A t-test was completed to test hypothesis two regrading differences between dental students and undergraduate students in student stress factors. It was found that dental students had significantly higher stress in regards to school and faculty (t=-6.337, p<0.001).

Results on prevalence of mental health symptoms and the association between student stress and mental health

A MANOVA and Kruskal-Wallis ANONVA were completed to test hypothesis one: there are differences in the stress, anxiety and depression levels among dental students, undergraduate university students and dental professionals. It was found that there were significant differences in the levels of stress between dental students and dental professionals, yielding an F ratio of 5.3 (p<0.01) (Table 11). Also it was found that there were significant differences in anxiety (x^2= 12.823, P=0.002) and depression (x^2 = 10.737, p=0.005) among all three groups, as shown in Table 12 below.

All other stressors were not significant (p>0.05) between the groups, indicating that the students felt similar amounts of perceived stress toward home and relationship, finance and future and time and workload. The results are shown in Table 10 below.

Table 11. Comparing stress between Dentist, Undergraduate student and Dental student. (Parametric variables) (N=152)

	Dentist (21)	Undergraduate Student (54)	Dental Student (77)	F	Post hoc.
Stress	9.6 (6.4)	13.37 (9.8)	16.75 (9.98)	5.3**	Dental student > Dentist **

**p<0.01.

Table 12. Kruskal-Wallis Test for determining differences in anxiety and depression between the groups (non-parametric variables) (N= 152)

	Dentist (n=21) Median (min,max)	Undergraduate Student (n=54) Median (min,max)	Dental Student (n=77) Median (min,max)	x^2	p-value
Anxiety	2 (0,14)	7 (0,28)	6 (0,36)	12.823	0.002
Depression	4 (0,14)	8 (0,34)	8 (0,40)	10.737	0.005

Table 13. Student stress as predictor of depression

Predictor variables	Regression coefficient (95% CI)	p-value
Student stress	0.130 (0.073-0.186)	**<0.001**
Age	-0.274 (-0.554-0.006)	**0.050**
Gender	0.594 (-1.263-2.452)	0.527
Individual/team sports	-0.303 (-0.877-0.271)	0.297
Leisure activities	-0.519 (-1.102-0.064)	0.080
Low GPA	1.744 (-0.956-4.445)	0.203
Later year of study	-1.446 (-3.316-0.424)	0.128
Prior tertiary study	-0.899 (-3.142-1.344)	0.428
Living with family	-2.491 (-4.446—0.536)	**0.013**

Correction coefficient (R)= .587

Adjusted R^2 = .269.

ANOVA F value = 4.577***.

Table 14. Student Stress as predictor of anxiety

Predictor variables	Regression coefficient (95% CI)	p-value
Student stress	0.138 (0.088-0.188)	**<0.001**
Age	-0.066 (-0.322-0.190)	0.609
Gender	1.344 (-0.303-2.991)	0.108
Team/individual sports	0.036 (-0.467-0.538)	0.889
Leisure activities	-0.180 (-0.691-0.331)	0.487
High GPA	-0.010 (-2.363-2.343)	0.993
Later year of study	-1.331 (-2.997-0.335)	0.116
Prior tertiary study	-0.326 (-2.281-1.629)	0.741
Living with family	-0.914 (-2.636-0.809)	0.295

Correlation coefficient (R)= 0.582.

Adjusted R^2 = 0.261.

ANOVA F value = 4.378***.

Linear regression models were run to determine the relationship between perceived student stress and aspects psychological dysfunction, namely depression, anxiety and stress. It was found that higher student stress score was positively associated with depression, (regression coefficient = 0.130, 95% CI= 0.073-0.186), anxiety (regression coefficient = 0.138, 95% CI= 0.088-0.188) and psychological stress (regression coefficient = 0.137, 95% CI= 0.088-0.186) and all associates were significant to p<0.001. The small confidence intervals indicate the accuracy of the association. The influence of confounding factors that were determined via Chi-square and t-test are described above and are also included in the models. The addition of the confounding factors did not alter the significance of the relationship between student stress and any aspect of psychological dysfunction. The Adjusted R^2 values for each model demonstrate that the variance accounted for by student stress and the confounders for each of the aspects of depression, anxiety and stress was 26.9%, 26.1% and 34.4% consecutively. This is an adequate amount of variance explained by the factors in each case. The results are shown below in Tables 13 to 15.

Table 15. Student Stress as predictor of psychological stress on DASS

Predictor variables	Regression coefficient (95% CI)	p-value
Student stress	0.137 (0.088-0.186)	**<0.001**
Age	-0.028 (-0.273-0.216)	0.819
Gender	2.914 (1.296-4.533)	**0.001**
Team/individual sports	0.151 (-0.305-0.652)	0.550
Leisure activities	-0.559 (-1.066- -0.051)	**0.031**
High GPA	-1.184 (-4.20400.506)	0.112
Lower year of study	-0.267 (-1.905-1.371)	0.747
Prior tertiary study	-1.277 (-3.253-0.700)	0.203
Living with family	-1.736 (-2.888-0.529)	0.174

Correlation coefficient (R)= 0.642.
Adjusted R^2 = 0.344.
ANOVA F value = 6.046***.
(For the above linear regressions *** indicates significance at the <0.001 level.).

Discussion

The current study endeavoured to gauge the levels of stress, anxiety and depression of dental students, using dentists and undergraduate students as relevant comparison groups. The levels of internal reliability of the DASS-21 questionnaire were similar to previous studies, indicating the consistency of the current sample (16).

In regards to the first hypothesis, which attempts to explore differences in psychological dysfunction between the three study groups, it was found that the hypothesis was partially supported. Dental students were significantly more stressed than dentists, though no significant difference was found with their comparison to undergraduate students. It was also found that there were significant difference between the groups for anxiety and depression. These results support the literature that suggests that dental students are under high amounts of psychological strain compared to dentists and other students (9,14).

From the results, the second hypothesis was also partially supported. Dental students were found to have significantly higher levels of stress regards to school and faculty. This may be due to the intense practical involvement of many parts of Dental School, when compared to a general university cohort. Dental students have the added pressure of learning practical clinical skills throughout their education, on top of an already heavy theoretical workload. The other factors all displayed a non-significant relationship between the groups. This finding demonstrates that university students actually share high levels of perceived stress, regardless of degree choice demonstrating the influence of the environmental factors associated with stress (2). This is supported by other studies of university students (7).

The results of this study also support the third hypothesis. Higher student stress is consistently associated with all aspects of psychological dysfunction. Firstly a strong predictive relationship was found between higher student stress and higher levels of depression. A protective influence of increasing age and living with family is evident in the stress-depression relationship in students. The protective effect of age is in accordance with other studies that suggest that age correlates negatively with depression (25). The apparent protective effect of living with family may suggest that increased family support is helpful in helping a student deal with stress issues so they don't led to depressive symptoms. Students stress also had a strong significant relationship with anxiety. The results showed that no confounding factors elicited a significant effect indicating an extremely predictive relationship between heightened student stress and high levels of anxiety.

Finally, the relationship between student stress and psychological stress was shown to be significantly positive. Gender also showed a significant positive relationship, indicating that females who are under stress were more likely to show symptoms of psychological stress. This is an interesting finding and may be possibly due to the influence of employed coping strategies. This is obviously an important issue for future investigations. It was also demonstrated that leisure activities such as shopping and going to the beach had a negative influence on the student stress-psychological stress relationship. This demonstrates the importance of 'switching off' and taking time out, so not to let perceived stress take its toll on and manifest as psychological symptoms.

Limitations

There are a number of limitations for the study. Shortfalls in any study may occur during sampling, data entry or within the actual study design itself. Selection bias may have been present in the current study. Though all efforts were made to include a wide range of participants, random sampling of participants from a sampling frame is the best way to reduce this type of error. Measurement bias of the self-report instrument may also have been present, though validity and reliability of the questionnaires has been verified in the current study as shown in appendix 1 and 2. There may also have been some response bias amongst the participants in the current study. Anonymity of the questionnaires attempted to keep this phenomenon to a minimum. Analysis bias involved in entering of data in SPSS is also a possibility in the current study. This may have skewed any final results, though checking and cleaning the data attempts to control this potential bias. It is also important to remember the possible influence of confounding factors in regards to the first two hypotheses. They cannot be directly entered into the models so their influence is unknown. The results should be interpreted with caution and in future, attempts at random sampling will hopefully ensure the demographic factors are similar between the groups.

Within the current study, data is only collected form a sub-sect of Australian dental and student populations and the generalizability of the results is limited. Efforts were made to represent all individuals within the cohort populations, though the sample will always be subject to sampling error (standard error). To improve generalizability of future results and to gain a better insight into student stress and mental health, a larger sample size from a broader range of universities and dental practices should be utilised. If possible, random sampling should also be employed. This reduces the standard error and may further aid in understanding psychological dysfunction in students and dental professionals.

Conclusion

In conclusion, it is apparent that dental students do suffer higher levels of stress in their university years than their graduates in the workplace. They also suffer higher levels of perceived stress in some factors, though it is made apparent in the study that the general university cohort is also suffering elevated levels of student stress and psychological dysfunction. A student's stress is strongly predictive of psychological dysfunction and this makes the implementation of stress reduction instruction an imperative part of tertiary education. Measures to reduce stress should be introduced and students should be educated in the importance of stress management in order to reduce the risk of physical and psychological morbidity. From the results of this investigation, future studies may now implement a randomised control trial to investigate the effects of an intervention program to combat psychological dysfunction in students.

Acknowledgments

Special thanks are due to all the students and staff at Griffith University Dental School and the dental clinics that took part. The authors would also like to thank Mrs S Peters for her continuous encouragement and help with sampling of the Dental professional population.

References

[1] Cohen S, Janicki-Deverts D, E. MG. Psychological stress and disease. JAMA 2007;298(14):1685-7.

[2] McEwen BS. Protective and damaging effects of stress mediators. N Engl J Med 1998;338(3):171-9.

[3] Polychronopoulou A, Divaris K. Dental students' perceived sources of stress: a multi-country study. J Dent Educ 2009;73(5):631-9.

[4] Gorter R, Freeman R, Hammen S, Murtomaa H, Blinkhorn A, Humphris G. Psychological stress and health in undergraduate dental students: fifth year outcomes compared with first year baseline results from five European dental schools. Eur J Dent Educ 2008;12(2):61-8.

[5] Naidu RS, Adams JS, Simeon D, Persad S. Sources of stress and psychological disturbance among dental students in the West Indies. J Dent Edu 2002;66(9):1021-30.

[6] Alzahem AM, van der Molen HT, Alaujan AH, Schmidt HG, Zamakhshary MH. Stress amongst dental students: a systematic review. Eur J Dent Edu 2011;15(1):8-18.

[7] Bayram N, Bilgel N. The prevalence and socio-demographic correlations of depression, anxiety and stress among a group of university students. Soc Psychiatry Psychiatr Epidemiol 2008;43(8):667-72.

[8] Hamaideh SH. Stressors and reactions to stressors among university students. Int J Soc Psychiat 2011;57(1):69-80.
[9] Murphy RJ, Gray SA, Sterling G, Reeves K, DuCette J. A comparative study of professional student stress. J Dent Edu 2009;73(3):328-37. .
[10] Alexander RE. Stress-related suicide by dentists and other health care workers. Fact or folklore? J Am Dent Assoc 2001;132(6):786-94.
[11] Sancho FM, Ruiz CN. Risk of suicide amongst dentists: myth or reality? Int Dent J 2010;60(6):411-8.
[12] Ayers KM, Thomson WM, Newton JT, Rich AM. Job stressors of New Zealand dentists and their coping strategies. Occup Med (Lond) 2008;58(4):275-81.
[13] Myers HL, Myers LB. 'It's difficult being a dentist': stress and health in the general dental practitioner. Br Dent J 2004;197(2):89-93.
[14] Newbury-Birch D, Lowry RJ, Kamali F. The changing patterns of drinking, illicit drug use, stress, anxiety and depression in dental students in a UK dental school: a longitudinal study. Br Dent J 2002;192(11):646-9.
[15] Lovibond SH, Lovibond PF. Manual for the Depression Anxiety Stress Scales. 2nd ed. Sydney: Sydney Psychology Foundation, 1995.
[16] Bentley MA, Crawford JM, Wilkins JR, Fernandez AR, Studnek JR. An Assessment of Depression, Anxiety, and Stress Among Nationally Certified EMS Professionals. Prehosp Emerg Care 2013, Epub 2013 Feb19.
[17] Tully PJ, Zajac IT, Venning AJ. The structure of anxiety and depression in a normative sample of younger and older Australian adolescents. J Abnorm Child Psychol 2009;37(5):717-26.
[18] Antony MM, Bieling PJ, Cox BJ, Enns MW, Swinson RP. Psychometric properties of the 42-item and 21-item versions of the Depression Anxiety Stress Scales in clinical groups and a community sample. Psychol Assessment 1998;10(2):176-81.
[19] Gloster AT, Rhoades HM, Novy D, Klotsche J, Senior A, Kunik M, et al. Psychometric properties of the Depression Anxiety and Stress Scale-21 in older primary care patients. J Affect Disord 2008;110(3):248-59.
[20] Henry JD, Crawford JR. The short-form version of the Depression Anxiety Stress Scales (DASS-21): construct validity and normative data in a large non-clinical sample. Br J Clin Psychol 2005;44(Pt 2):227-39. 21. Sinclair SJ, Siefert CJ, Slavin-Mulford JM, Stein MB, Renna M, Blais MA. Psychometric evaluation and normative data for the depression, anxiety, and stress scales-21 (DASS-21) in a nonclinical sample of U.S. adults. Eval Health Prof 2012;35(3):259-79.
[21] Garbee WH, Jr., Zucker SB, Selby GR. Perceived sources of stress among dental students. J Am Dent Assoc 1980;100(6):853-7.
[22] Sanders AE, Lushington K. Sources of stress for Australian dental students. J Dent Educ 1999;63(9):688-97.
[23] Westerman GH, Grandy TG, Ocanto RA, Erskine CG. Perceived sources of stress in the dental school environment. J Dent Educ 1993;57(3):225-31.
[24] Christensen H, Jorm AF, Mackinnon AJ, Korten AE, Jacomb PA, Henderson AS, et al. Age differences in depression and anxiety symptoms: a structural equation modelling analysis of data from a general population sample. Psychol Med 1999;29(2):325-39.

In: Health Promotion
Editors: J. Sun, N. Buys, J. Merrick

ISBN: 978-1-62257-870-2

Chapter IX

Effect of green tea consumption on obesity and hypertension: A systematic review protocol

Saman Khalesi*[*,1], Jing Sun, PhD[1] and Nicholas Buys, PhD[2]
[1]School of Public Health and Griffith Health Institute, Griffith University, Gold Coast Campus, Parkland, Australia
[2]School of Human Services and Social Work, and Griffith Health Institute, Griffith University, Parkland, Gold Coast, Australia

Abstract

Green tea is a healthy drink and evidence of its positive effect on both obesity and hypertension is emerging. This review protocol is concerned with the efficacy of green tea consumption in improving health status of people with obesity and hypertension. Interventional randomized or non-randomized studies, as well as cross sectional studies, with a focus on the effect of green tea consumption on obesity and/or hypertension will be

[*] *Correspondence:* Saman Khalesi, Griffith Health Institute and School of Public Health, Gold Coast Campus, Parkland, Q4222 Australia. E-mail: saman.khalesitaharoom@griffithuni.edu.au.

identified. Literature will be searched by two authors independently through Medline, PubMed, Scopus and Cochrane library.
All articles from January 2003 to end of May 2013, which meet the inclusion/exclusion criteria, will be studied. Human studies analyzing the effect of green tea consumption on either obesity or hypertension or both, or respective indicators (oriental tea, anthropometry, abdominal fat, central fat, body mass index, blood lipid profile, metabolic syndrome, high blood pressure, systolic blood pressure and diastolic blood pressure, waist circumference and waist hip ratio) will be included. Study of indicators will only be included, if the endpoint data reports an association or correlation with obesity and/or hypertension. Only studies with focus on green tea, oriental tea or green tea extract or its catechins will be included. Studies with artificial catechins or catechins from sources other than green tea will not be included. Search terms will include green tea, *Camellia sinensis*, green tea extract, green tea catechins, green tea supplements with obesity, overweight, abdominal fat, central fat, metabolic syndrome, hypertension, blood pressure, anthropometry, waist circumference, waist/hip ratio and blood lipid profile.

Introduction

Obesity has become one of the world's most epidemic diseases with more than 1.4 billion people either obese or overweight (1). Obesity is now the fifth leading risk of all death in the world and a main cause of cardiovascular disease, diabetes, and stroke (1). Obesity is characterized by a body mass index (BMI) of 30 or more and overweight by a BMI of more than 25 and less than 30 (2). In Australia three out of five adults are either overweight or obese and the prevalence of obesity among males, 18 years and older, increased from 57.5% in 2001 to 62.8% in 2007-08 and among females, 18 years and older, increased from 42.2% in 2001 to 47.6% in 2007-08 (3). Hypertension, another epidemic disease, is also a major cause of cardiovascular disease and stroke. In the United States (US) the prevalence of hypertension among people 18 years and older was 28.6% in 2009-2010(4). There have been some recent advances in the treatment of hypertension. However, approximately two thirds of hypertensive people in the US have not controlled their high blood pressure levels (5). In 2005, 14% of people age 45-54 and 41% of those over 75 had hypertension in Australia (6).

Tea is the most frequently consumed beverage around the world after water (7). There is increasing evidence to demonstrate that green tea may have an effect on preventing hypertension and obesity. Green tea is made from the steamed and dried leaves of the *Camellia sinensis* plant. It is a widely consumed beverage containing healthy phenolic components, which have anti-oxidative effects on the body. Numerous studies have been published on green tea and its health benefits on lipid profile (8,9) blood glucose level (10), and cancer (11,12). The effectiveness of green tea in improving hypertension or weight reduction and management, along with other complications, has been investigated in both animal and human studies (13-15). However, there is no systematic review of the literature summarizing the association between green tea and obesity and hypertension. The present study aims to undertake this review as a step towards a future intervention study.

Study objectives

The primary aim of this systematic review is to summarize and examine literature on the association between green tea consumption and obesity and hypertension at population level. Following this it is expected that green tea consumption may be found to have effect on lowering blood pressure level and body weight and improvement of blood lipid profile.

Study questions

In this systematic review the following questions are addressed:

1. Does green tea have an impact on reducing obesity? If so, is the effect significant?
2. Does green tea have an impact on reducing hypertension? If so, is the effect significant? What is the optimal intake of green tea consumption to provide the greatest impact on obesity and/or hypertension?

Design

To address the study aim and questions a comprehensive literature search will be undertaken. Human trials that assess the effect of green tea on obesity or hypertension will be reviewed, including randomized parallel interventions and uncontrolled before-and-after studies. The reporting of the review will follow the "Preferred Reporting Items for Systematic Reviews and Meta-Analysis: the PRISMA statement" (16). All methodologies in studies reviewed will be assessed using the validated quality checklist developed by Downs and Black (17).

Search methods

Literature on green tea consumption and its impact, for the period January 2003 to the end of May 2013, will be identified using electronic databases of Medline, PubMed, Scopus and Cochrane Library (CENTERAL). Grey literature (publications issued by government, academia and industry or uncontrolled by commercial publishing interests) (18) will be searched through the OpenGrey database. Search terms are detailed in Table 1.

Database searches, scanning and screening of articles will be undertaken independently by two authors. Both authors will follow the eligibility criteria to include or exclude articles. In case of any disagreement, the matter will be resolved through discussion. A third author will be involved in decision making if consensus cannot be reached between the first two reviewers.

Table 1. Search Terms

Search String	AND
Green tea	Obesity
Camellia sinensis	Hypertension
Catechins	Overweight
Green tea extract	Body Mass Index
Green tea supplement	Abdominal fat
Oriental tea	Central fat
	Waist circumference
	Waist hip ratio
	Anthropometry
	Metabolic syndrome
	Blood lipid profile
	Blood pressure
	Triglyceride
	Serum cholesterol
	Blood glucose
	High density lipoprotein
	Low density lipoprotein

All combination of search terms would be considered and run through the search engine. All article citations related to the search combination would be saved through EndNote, regardless of duplications, for further screening. Screening of saved articles will begin by removing duplicates and reviewing the titles at first stage and going through the abstract and complete article at next stages. Choosing articles would be by considering eligibilities and inclusion criteria.

Eligible studies

All human randomized interventional studies which address green tea consumption with obesity or hypertension or both would be included. Only literature published in English language will be considered. Human trials which focus on green tea consumption or its catechins, extract or supplements will be studied. Artificial catechins or catechins extracted from sources other than green tea will be excluded.

Studies of the effect of green tea on lipid profile will only be included if the reported end point data is on obesity and/or hypertension or the findings show correlations or associations between consumption and obesity and/or hypertension.

Studies which fail to address the dosage and frequency of green tea consumption or fail to mention intervention period will be excluded. The number of excluded studies and the reasons of exclusion will be noted.

Data extraction

Data will be extracted by the two reviewers from the included articles. In the case of any missing data, vague results or needs for complementary data, the corresponding author of the article will be contacted to clarify the information. For the dosage of green tea the preferential unit of reporting is gram of green tea. Units of dosage other than gram of green tea (e.g. milliliter, milligram, or number of cups), would be calculated to the nearest approximate gram of solid green tea. The intended data to be extracted from articles is mention in the table 2.

Table 2. Components of data extraction

Intended data to be extracted from articles
- General information of the paper (title, authors, publication details, year of publication, etc.)
- Study type (randomized controlled trials, cohort, etc.)
- Population characteristics (demographic, geographical settings, size of population, health status, etc.)
- Intervention characteristics (location, length of study, dosage and frequency of green tea consumption, number of dropouts, etc.)
- Eligibility (inclusion and exclusion criteria of the study)
- Result and outcome (changes, mean differences, odd ratio, *p*-value, etc.)
- Follow up data (period, results, if available)
- Adverse effect (if applicable)
- Limitations (if applicable)
- Important notes or conclusions of authors

Methodology quality assessment

The quality of eligible articles, in case of their methodology, will be assessed using a 32- score quality checklist developed by Downs and Black (17). The checklist was developed for both randomized controlled trials and non-randomized studies. To interpret the scoring system we will follow the method used by Harrison et al. (19), where scores higher than 12 would be considered good quality papers. Data may be considered from papers with lower scores if the number of selected articles is inadequate. The scoring scale developed by Downs and Black (17) consists of 27 items with total of 32 scores. The sections and items to be assessed in each article are mentioned in Table 3. The scoring will be carried out by both reviewers.

Data analysis methods

Data will be presented in tabular and narrative form. Information on year, setting, population, intervention, outcome and quality of studies will be presented in tables. Outcome measures of Relative risk (RR) or odds ratio (OR) of included studies with confidence interval of 95%, with or without green tea consumption, will be reported in tables as well. Where necessary, an attempt to calculate the quantity of missed value will be made. A footnote will document how the value is calculated.

Table 3. The measuring sections and items to assess articles' quality of methodology

Measuring sections	Measuring items
Reporting	Clear hypothesis, aim and objective
	Clear described main outcomes
	Clear described characteristics of patients
	Clear described of intervention
	Clear described confounder distribution among groups
	Clear described main outcomes
	Provided estimates of random variability in data of main outcome
	Reported adverse events of the intervention
	Described characteristics of patients lost to follow-up
	Reported actual probability value for main outcome
External validity	Subjects asked to participate represented the entire population of recruitment
	Subjects actually participated represented the entire population of recruitment
	Study treatment environment represented the entire population treatment environment
Internal validity-bias	Study attempted to blind study the subject through intervention
	Study attempted to blind those measuring main outcomes
	Clear in using "data dredging", if applicable
	Analysis adjusted for different length of follow-up, if applicable
	Appropriate statistical approaches to assess outcomes
	Reliable compliance with the intervention
Internal validity-confounding (selection bias)	Accurate outcome measures
	Participants in different groups recruited from same population
	Participants in different groups recruited over the same time period
	Randomization of participants into study groups
	Concealed randomization until completion of recruitment
Power	Adequate adjusted confounding in the analysis
	Accounted losses of patients to follow-up
	Sufficient power of study to detect clinically important effect, when the probability of chance is less than 5%

Reporting of results

The results of the systematic review will be reported following guidelines set by the Preferred Reporting Items for Systematic Review (PRISMA) study group (16). All papers extracted data will be presented in tables. Odds ratio, *p*-value and mean differences of included studies will be presented in tables as well. A narrative comparative approach will discuss the finding of each paper and the similarities/differences of the results of selected papers will be discussed. Finally the guideline for green tea interventions and possible improving effect on obesity and hypertension will be discussed.

Expected outcomes and significance of study

Through this study we expect to understand the effect of green tea consumption on improvement of health status of people with obesity and/or hypertension. It is anticipated that a correlation between dosage of green tea consumption and its effectiveness and correlation between length of green team consumption and its effectiveness will be found. Moreover, the best method of consuming green tea (as tea, supplement or extract) as well as the most influenced age group and gender would be expected from this review. As the secondary outcome we anticipate finding any association between green tea consumption and or indicators (blood lipid profile, waist circumference and etc.). Although green tea has been used in many interventional studies and clinical trials for treatment of obesity and hypertension, the effectiveness of the green tea usage and the dosage related information is not clear. This systematic review of literature may provide reliable information on green tea consumption for practitioners or researchers dealing with obesity and hypertension. It may be helpful for dieticians planning diets for obese or hypertensive patients as well. Moreover, it can provide a guideline for industries dealing with green tea extract or supplements to improve obesity or hypertensive conditions.

Ethics and dissemination

Our systematic review is to evaluate the effectiveness of green tea on obesity and hypertension base on reviewing literature and previous studies. As no primary data collection or intervention would be undertaken, ethical clearance will not be required. The review protocol however, has been registered with the International Prospective Register of Systematic Review (PROSPERO) with registration number CRD42013004720. The result of the review will be submitted for publication in peer reviewed journals. This study will begin in June, 2013, with reporting of study findings by September, 2013.

Limitations

The limitations of this systematic review will be as follow: 1) publications will be restricted to those English, thereby potentially limiting the range of studies reviewed; 2) if any essential data is missing, the corresponding author will be contacted. However poor or incomplete reports of study design, patient population, and intervention may impact the quality of interpretation of findings (20); 3) as a review will include a wide range of studies, there will not be any homogeneity between populations in term of patient demographic variables, diet or other characteristics. Although this may affect the generalization of our interpretations, we will attempt to differentiate our reporting base on various characteristics.

References

[1] Obesity and overweight. Fact sheet n 311 [database on the Internet]. WHO 2012.

[2] Obesity: preventing and managing the global epidemic. Report of a WHO consultation report series 894 [database on the Internet]. WHO 2000.

[3] Gender Indicators. cat no.4125.0 [database on the Internet]. ABS 2012.

[4] Ogden CL, Carroll MD, Kit BK, Flegal KM. Prevalence of obesity in the United States, 2009-2010. Washington, DC: US Department of Health and Human Services, Centers for Disease Control and Prevention, National Center for Health Statistics, 2012.

[5] Hajjar I, Kotchen JM, Kotchen TA. Hypertension: trends in prevalence, incidence, and control. Annu Rev Public Health 2006;27(1):465-90.

[6] Australia Bureau of Statistics, Australia, 2004-05. cat. no.4364.0 [database on the Internet]. ABS 2006.

[7] Schneider C, Segre T. Green tea: potential health benefits. Am Fam Physician 2009;79(7):591-4.

[8] Erba D, Riso P, Bordoni A, Foti P, Biagi PL, Testolin G. Effectiveness of moderate green tea consumption on antioxidative status and plasma lipid profile in humans. J Nutr Biochem 2005;16(3):144.

[9] Maron DJ, Lu GP, Cai NS, Wu ZG, Li YH, Chen H, et al. Cholesterol-lowering effect of a theaflavin-enriched green tea extract: a randomized controlled trial. Arch Intern Med 2003;163(12):1448.

[10] Maruyama K, Iso H, Sasaki S, Fukino Y. The association between concentrations of green tea and blood glucose levels. J Clin Biochem Nutr 2009;44(1):41.

[11] Mu LN, Lu QY, Yu SZ, Jiang QW, Cao W, You NC, et al. Green tea drinking and multigenetic index on the risk of stomach cancer in a Chinese population. Int J Cancer 2005;116(6):972-83.

[12] Sun C-L, Yuan J-M, Koh W-P, Mimi CY. Green tea, black tea and breast cancer risk: a meta-analysis of epidemiological studies. Carcinogenesis 2006;27(7):1310-5.

[13] Antonello M, Montemurro D, Bolognesi M, Di Pascoli M, Piva A, Grego F, et al. Prevention of Hypertension, Cardiovascular Damage and Endothelial Dysfunction with Green Tea Extracts. Am J Hypertens 2007;20(12):1321-8.

[14] Auvichayapat P, Prapochanung M, Tunkamnerdthai O, Sripanidkulchai B-o, Auvichayapat N, Thinkhamrop B, et al. Effectiveness of green tea on weight reduction in obese Thais: A randomized, controlled trial. Physiol Behav 2008;93(3):486-91.

[15] Nagao T, Hase T, Tokimitsu I. A green tea extract high in catechins reduces body fat and cardiovascular risks in humans. Obesity 2007;15(6):1473-83.

[16] Moher D, Liberati A, Tetzlaff J, Altman DG. Preferred reporting items for systematic reviews and meta-analyses: the PRISMA statement. Ann Intern Med 2009;151(4):264-9.

[17] Downs SH, Black N. The feasibility of creating a checklist for the assessment of the methodological quality both of randomised and non-randomised studies of health care interventions. J Epidemiol Community Health 1998;52(6):377-84.

[18] Bowling A. Research methods in health: investigating health and health services. Maidenhead: Open University Press, 2009.

[19] Harrison RA, Siminoski K, Vethanayagam D, Majumdar SR. Osteoporosis-Related Kyphosis and Impairments in Pulmonary Function: A Systematic Review. J Bone Miner Res 2007;22(3):447-57.

[20] Glasziou P, Meats E, Heneghan C, Shepperd S. What is missing from descriptions of treatment in trials and reviews? BMJ (Clinical research ed) 2008;336(7659):1472-4.

SECTION THREE: ACKNOWLEDGMENTS

Chapter X

About the authors

Jing Sun, PhD, is a senior lecturer of School of Public Health at Griffith University in Australia. She has bachelor, master degree in education psychology and PhD degree in Neuropsychology. Her research interests are in child and adolescent health, employee's mental health, mental health promotion, biostatistics and epidemiology, with a particular focus on the mental health, multilevel and statistical modelling development, primary prevention in chronic diseases in national and international context. She has published extensively in international journals in areas of mental health promotion, entrepreneurships, prefrontal lobe functioning in infants, smoking cessation program, community singing program, and resilience based program. Email: j.sun@griffith.edu.au

Nicholas Buys, BA(Hons), MSc, PhD, Professor Nicholas Buys is a Dean in Teaching and Leaning in Health Faculty at Griffith University, Australia. He has bachelor degree in psychology, and master and PhD degree in human rehabilitation. His research interests range from human rehabilitation, mental health, mental health promotion, to population health. He has published widely in international journals in areas of mental health promotion in Australian Aboriginal and Torres Strait Islander people, social inequality in disadvantaged population, social inclusion, entrepreneurship, risk health behavior, and primary prevention of chronic disease. E-mail: n.buys@griffith.edu.au

Joav Merrick, MD, MMedSci, DMSc, is professor of pediatrics, child health and human development affiliated with Kentucky Children's Hospital, University of Kentucky, Lexington, United States and the Division of Pediatrics, Hadassah Hebrew University Medical Center, Mt Scopus

Campus, Jerusalem, Israel, the medical director of the Health Services, Division for Intellectual and Developmental Disabilities, Ministry of Social Affairs and Social Services, Jerusalem, the founder and director of the National Institute of Child Health and Human Development in Israel. Numerous publications in the field of pediatrics, child health and human development, rehabilitation, intellectual disability, disability, health, welfare, abuse, advocacy, quality of life and prevention. Received the Peter Sabroe Child Award for outstanding work on behalf of Danish Children in 1985 and the International LEGO-Prize ("The Children's Nobel Prize") for an extraordinary contribution towards improvement in child welfare and well-being in 1987. E-mail: jmerrick@zahav.net.il

Chapter XI

About Griffith Health, Griffith University, Queensland, Australia

Griffith Health at Griffith University has first-rate education programs with leading award-winning teachers and industry partners in order to help build healthy and happy communities.

Griffith Health provides:

- Undergraduate programs
- Postgraduate programs
- Research programs
- Continuing education programs

Griffith Health's high quality, innovative education programs range from the foundation health sciences to professional and clinical disciplines. Our teaching programs are supported by our world-class health research centres. Griffith Health is one of Australia's largest health faculties with over 6500 full time students enjoying state-of-the-art learning facilities and the most up-to-date teaching programs.

We are committed to achieving excellence in public health research and postgraduate research training, and to developing high quality undergraduate and postgraduate courses of relevance to a changing society and recognised by professional bodies and accreditation authorities. Our distinctive socio-ecological approach integrates public, environmental and occupational health concerns with policy and service management considerations.

The Bachelor of Public Health is a multi-disciplinary three-year program that provides the knowledge and skills to work in a wide range of public health professions. Integrating knowledge and practice from a range of fields such as environmental health, health promotion, and nutrition and dietetics. Focussing on the systems and practices that shape the health of nations, communities and individuals and the environments in which they live, work and take their leisure.

Issues that help determine quality of life are investigated, such as globalisation, technology, environmental degradation and population trends, lifestyle and nutrition, control of existing and emerging communicable diseases, industry pollution management, food and drug safety.

Contact:
Griffith Health
E-mail: health@griffith.edu.au

Chapter XII

About the National Institute of Child Health and Human Development in Israel

The National Institute of Child Health and Human Development (NICHD) in Israel was established in 1998 as a virtual institute under the auspicies of the Medical Director, Ministry of Social Affairs and Social Services in order to function as the research arm for the Office of the Medical Director. In 1998 the National Council for Child Health and Pediatrics, Ministry of Health and in 1999 the Director General and Deputy Director General of the Ministry of Health endorsed the establishment of the NICHD.

Mission

The mission of a National Institute for Child Health and Human Development in Israel is to provide an academic focal point for the scholarly interdisciplinary study of child life, health, public health, welfare, disability, rehabilitation, intellectual disability and related aspects of human development. This mission includes research, teaching, clinical work, information and public service activities in the field of child health and human development.

Service and academic activities

Over the years many activities became focused in the south of Israel due to collaboration with various professionals at the Faculty of Health Sciences (FOHS) at the Ben Gurion University of the Negev (BGU). Since 2000 an affiliation with the Zusman Child Development Center at the Pediatric Division of Soroka University Medical Center has resulted in collaboration around the establishment of the Down Syndrome Clinic at that center. In 2002 a full course on "Disability" was established at the Recanati School for Allied Professions in the Community, FOHS, BGU and in 2005 collaboration was started with the Primary Care Unit of the faculty and disability became part of the master of public health course on "Children and society". In the academic year 2005-2006 a one semester course on "Aging with disability" was started as part of the master of science program in gerontology in our collaboration with the Center for Multidisciplinary Research in Aging. In 2010 collaborations with the Division of Pediatrics, Hadassah Medical Center, Hebrew University, Jerusalem, Israel.

Research activities

The affiliated staff have over the years published work from projects and research activities in this national and international collaboration. In the year 2000 the International Journal of Adolescent Medicine and Health and in 2005 the International Journal on Disability and Human development of De Gruyter Publishing House (Berlin and New York), in the year 2003 the TSW-Child Health and Human Development and in 2006 the TSW-Holistic Health and Medicine of the Scientific World Journal (New York and Kirkkonummi, Finland), all peer-reviewed international journals were affiliated with the National Institute of Child Health and Human Development. From 2008 also the International Journal of Child Health and Human Development (Nova Science, New York), the International Journal of Child and Adolescent Health (Nova Science) and the Journal of Pain Management (Nova Science) affiliated and from 2009 the International Public Health Journal (Nova Science) and Journal of Alternative Medicine Research (Nova Science).

National collaborations

Nationally the NICHD works in collaboration with the Faculty of Health Sciences, Ben Gurion University of the Negev; Department of Physical Therapy, Sackler School of Medicine, Tel Aviv University; Autism Center, Assaf HaRofeh Medical Center; National Rett and PKU Centers at Chaim Sheba Medical Center, Tel HaShomer; Department of Physiotherapy, Haifa University; Department of Education, Bar Ilan University, Ramat Gan, Faculty of Social Sciences and Health Sciences; College of Judea and Samaria in Ariel and in 2011 affiliation with Center for Pediatric Chronic Diseases and Center for Down Syndrome, Department of Pediatrics, Hadassah-Hebrew University Medical Center, Mount Scopus Campus, Jerusalem.

International collaborations

Internationally with the Department of Disability and Human Development, College of Applied Health Sciences, University of Illinois at Chicago; Strong Center for Developmental Disabilities, Golisano Children's Hospital at Strong, University of Rochester School of Medicine and Dentistry, New York; Centre on Intellectual Disabilities, University of Albany, New York; Centre for Chronic Disease Prevention and Control, Health Canada, Ottawa; Chandler Medical Center and Children's Hospital, Kentucky Children's Hospital, Section of Adolescent Medicine, University of Kentucky, Lexington; Chronic Disease Prevention and Control Research Center, Baylor College of Medicine, Houston, Texas; Division of Neuroscience, Department of Psychiatry, Columbia University, New York; Institute for the Study of Disadvantage and Disability, Atlanta; Center for Autism and Related Disorders, Department Psychiatry, Children's Hospital Boston, Boston; Department of Paediatrics, Child Health and Adolescent Medicine, Children's Hospital at Westmead, Westmead, Australia; International Centre for the Study of Occupational and Mental Health, Düsseldorf, Germany; Centre for Advanced Studies in Nursing, Department of General Practice and Primary Care, University of Aberdeen, Aberdeen, United Kingdom; Quality of Life Research Center, Copenhagen, Denmark; Nordic School of Public Health, Gottenburg, Sweden, Scandinavian Institute of Quality of Working Life, Oslo, Norway; Centre for Quality of Life of the Hong Kong Institute of Asia-Pacific Studies and School of Social Work, Chinese University, Hong Kong.

Targets

Our focus is on research, international collaborations, clinical work, teaching and policy in health, disability and human development and to establish the NICHD as a permanent institute at one of the residential care centers for persons with intellectual disability in Israel in order to conduct model research and together with the four university schools of public health/medicine in Israel establish a national master and doctoral program in disability and human development at the institute to secure the next generation of professionals working in this often non-prestigious/low-status field of work.

Contact:

Joav Merrick, MD, DMSc
Professor of Pediatrics, Child Health and Human Development
Medical Director, Health Services, Division for Intellectual and Developmental Disabilities, Ministry of Social Affairs and Social Services, POB 1260, IL-91012 Jerusalem, Israel.
E-mail: jmerrick@zahav.net.il

Chapter XIII

About the book series "Health and human development"

Health and human development is a book series with publications from a multidisciplinary group of researchers, practitioners and clinicians for an international professional forum interested in the broad spectrum of health and human development. Books already published:

- Merrick J, Omar HA, eds. Adolescent behavior research. International perspectives. New York: Nova Science, 2007.
- Kratky KW. Complementary medicine systems: Comparison and integration. New York: Nova Science, 2008.
- Schofield P, Merrick J, eds. Pain in children and youth. New York: Nova Science, 2009.
- Greydanus DE, Patel DR, Pratt HD, Calles Jr JL, eds. Behavioral pediatrics, 3 ed. New York: Nova Science, 2009.
- Ventegodt S, Merrick J, eds. Meaningful work: Research in quality of working life. New York: Nova Science, 2009.
- Omar HA, Greydanus DE, Patel DR, Merrick J, eds. Obesity and adolescence. A public health concern. New York: Nova Science, 2009.
- Lieberman A, Merrick J, eds. Poverty and children. A public health concern. New York: Nova Science, 2009.
- Goodbread J. Living on the edge. The mythical, spiritual and philosophical roots of social marginality. New York: Nova Science, 2009.

- Bennett DL, Towns S, Elliot E, Merrick J, eds. Challenges in adolescent health: An Australian perspective. New York: Nova Science, 2009.
- Schofield P, Merrick J, eds. Children and pain. New York: Nova Science, 2009.
- Sher L, Kandel I, Merrick J, eds. Alcohol-related cognitive disorders: Research and clinical perspectives. New York: Nova Science, 2009.
- Anyanwu EC. Advances in environmental health effects of toxigenic mold and mycotoxins. New York: Nova Science, 2009.
- Bell E, Merrick J, eds. Rural child health. International aspects. New York: Nova Science, 2009.
- Dubowitz H, Merrick J, eds. International aspects of child abuse and neglect. New York: Nova Science, 2010.
- Shahtahmasebi S, Berridge D. Conceptualizing behavior: A practical guide to data analysis. New York: Nova Science, 2010.
- Wernik U. Chance action and therapy. The playful way of changing. New York: Nova Science, 2010.
- Omar HA, Greydanus DE, Patel DR, Merrick J, eds. Adolescence and chronic illness. A public health concern. New York: Nova Science, 2010.
- Patel DR, Greydanus DE, Omar HA, Merrick J, eds. Adolescence and sports. New York: Nova Science, 2010.
- Shek DTL, Ma HK, Merrick J, eds. Positive youth development: Evaluation and future directions in a Chinese context. New York: Nova Science, 2010.
- Shek DTL, Ma HK, Merrick J, eds. Positive youth development: Implementation of a youth program in a Chinese context. New York: Nova Science, 2010.
- Omar HA, Greydanus DE, Tsitsika AK, Patel DR, Merrick J, eds. Pediatric and adolescent sexuality and gynecology: Principles for the primary care clinician. New York: Nova Science, 2010.
- Chow E, Merrick J, eds. Advanced cancer. Pain and quality of life. New York: Nova Science, 2010.
- Latzer Y, Merrick, J, Stein D, eds. Understanding eating disorders. Integrating culture, psychology and biology. New York: Nova Science, 2010.
- Sahgal A, Chow E, Merrick J, eds. Bone and brain metastases: Advances in research and treatment. New York: Nova Science, 2010.
- Postolache TT, Merrick J, eds. Environment, mood disorders and suicide. New York: Nova Science, 2010.

- Maharajh HD, Merrick J, eds. Social and cultural psychiatry experience from the Caribbean Region. New York: Nova Science, 2010.
- Mirsky J. Narratives and meanings of migration. New York: Nova Science, 2010.
- Harvey PW. Self-management and the health care consumer. New York: Nova Science, 2011.
- Ventegodt S, Merrick J. Sexology from a holistic point of view. New York: Nova Science, 2011.
- Ventegodt S, Merrick J. Principles of holistic psychiatry: A textbook on holistic medicine for mental disorders. New York: Nova Science, 2011.
- Greydanus DE, Calles Jr JL, Patel DR, Nazeer A, Merrick J, eds. Clinical aspects of psychopharmacology in childhood and adolescence. New York: Nova Science, 2011.
- Bell E, Seidel BM, Merrick J, eds. Climate change and rural child health. New York: Nova Science, 2011.
- Bell E, Zimitat C, Merrick J, eds. Rural medical education: Practical strategies. New York: Nova Science, 2011.
- Latzer Y, Tzischinsky. The dance of sleeping and eating among adolescents: Normal and pathological perspectives. New York: Nova Science, 2011.
- Deshmukh VD. The astonishing brain and holistic consciousness: Neuroscience and Vedanta perspectives. New York: Nova Science, 2011.
- Bell E, Westert GP, Merrick J, eds. Translational research for primary healthcare. New York: Nova Science, 2011.
- Shek DTL, Sun RCF, Merrick J, eds. Drug abuse in Hong Kong: Development and evaluation of a prevention program. New York: Nova Science, 2011.
- Ventegodt S, Hermansen TD, Merrick J. Human Development: Biology from a holistic point of view. New York: Nova Science, 2011.
- Ventegodt S, Merrick J. Our search for meaning in life. New York: Nova Science, 2011.
- Caron RM, Merrick J, eds. Building community capacity: Minority and immigrant populations. New York: Nova Science, 2012.
- Klein H, Merrick J, eds. Human immunodeficiency virus (HIV) research: Social science aspects. New York: Nova Science, 2012.
- Lutzker JR, Merrick J, eds. Applied public health: Examining multifaceted Social or ecological problems and child maltreatment. New York: Nova Science, 2012.

- Chemtob D, Merrick J, eds. AIDS and tuberculosis: Public health aspects. New York: Nova Science, 2012.
- Ventegodt S, Merrick J. Textbook on evidence-based holistic mind-body medicine: Basic principles of healing in traditional Hippocratic medicine. New York: Nova Science, 2012.
- Ventegodt S, Merrick J. Textbook on evidence-based holistic mind-body medicine: Holistic practice of traditional Hippocratic medicine. New York: Nova Science, 2012.
- Ventegodt S, Merrick J. Textbook on evidence-based holistic mind-body medicine: Healing the mind in traditional Hippocratic medicine. New York: Nova Science, 2012.
- Ventegodt S, Merrick J. Textbook on evidence-based holistic mind-body medicine: Sexology and traditional Hippocratic medicine. New York: Nova Science, 2012.
- Ventegodt S, Merrick J. Textbook on evidence-based holistic mind-body medicine: Research, philosophy, economy and politics of traditional Hippocratic medicine. New York: Nova Science, 2012.
- Caron RM, Merrick J, eds. Building community capacity: Skills and principles. New York: Nova Science, 2012.
- Lemal M, Merrick J, eds. Health risk communication. New York: Nova Science, 2012.
- Ventegodt S, Merrick J. Textbook on evidence-based holistic mind-body medicine: Basic philosophy and ethics of traditional Hippocratic medicine. New York: Nova Science, 2013.
- Caron RM, Merrick J, eds. Building community capacity: Case examples from around the world. New York: Nova Science, 2013.
- Steele RE. Managed care in a public setting. New York: Nova Science, 2013.
- Srabstein JC, Merrick J, eds. Bullying: A public health concern. New York: Nova Science, 2013.
- Thavarajah N, Pulenzas N, Lechner B, Chow E, Merrick J, eds. Advanced cancer: Managing symptoms and quality of life. New York: Nova Science, 2013.
- Stein D, Latzer Y, eds. Treatment and recovery of eating disorders. New York: Nova Science, 2013.
- Sun J, Buys N, Merrick J. Health promotion: Community singing as a vehicle to promote health. New York: Nova Science, 2013.

Contact:
Professor Joav Merrick, MD, MMedSci, DMSc
Medical Director, Health Services
Division for Intellectual and Developmental Disabailities
Ministry of Social Affairs and Social Services
POBox 1260, IL-91012 Jerusalem, Israel
E-mail: jmerrick@zahav.net.il

Index

A

D

E

F

G

H

I

J

L

N

O

P

Q

R

S

Y